Moving Away From Diets

by

Karin Kratina, MA, RD, LD
Nancy King, MS, RD, CDE
Dayle Hayes, MS, RD, LD

Helm Publishing
Lake Dallas, TX

Disclaimer: Decisions regarding health care and medical nutrition therapy should be undertaken after a careful review of an individual's health status, medical history, and current diagnosis. Based on these factors, the nondiet approach described in this book may not be appropriate for some individuals. Questions regarding the suitability of any nutrition care plan are best addressed by the individual client in consultation with his or her health care provider, nutrition therapist, and other members of the health care team.

Moving Away From Diets, third printing

Cover design: The Wyatt Group
Copyediting: Jacqueline Marcus, MS, RD, FADA, Peggy Leslie, and Harvey Mueller
Editor: Kathy King, RD, LD
Printer/ binder: Sheridan Books
Copyright 1996, 1999, 2002 by Helm Publishing

For information or to order books, camera-ready handouts, or study guides, call, fax, or write:

Helm Publishing
P.O. Box 2105
Lake Dallas, TX 75065
phone (940) 497-3558   fax (940) 497-2927
www.helmpublishing.com

ISBN 0-9631033-5-0

TABLE OF CONTENTS

Foreword

Clinical studies and clinical observations support the association of weight loss to improvement of hypertension, diabetes, and hyperlipidemia. Accordingly, many clinical societies advocate weight loss as the first tier of treatment of significantly obese patients.

After over 24 years of treating thousands of patients with diet-sensitive diseases, I have come to the conclusion that diets do not work. Initially, my internist colleagues and I tried the still common practices of encouraging calorie restriction and slowing the eating process. The four month follow-up response to such a treatment revealed half the patients lost weight and half the patients gained. No change.

Twenty years ago, I introduced a dietitian to my outpatient practice. She had more time to spend with the patient, was more skilled in behavior modification, and was able to tailor the patient's food choices closer to lower calorie food. The average weight loss was 14 pounds in four months; unfortunately, all the weight was regained in the ensuing year.

Not to give in to failure, I introduced the combined treatment of the dietitian and doctor, more frequent visits, and a metered liquid diet. Although our initial approach was successful, an average of 50 pounds lost in 5 months, our three year follow-up revealed 60 pounds were regained. In other words, the liquid diet program caused a 10 pound weight gain!

After this failure, I became disillusioned with the treatment of obesity. I was only partly comforted to know that other researchers suffered the same results. Diets did not work.

Further inspection revealed that patients were adversely affected by dieting. A number of patients failed to return for medical care, presumably because of their failure to lose weight. Others were consumed by continued dieting efforts with much of their waking hours spent on dieting thoughts. The cost of the various failed programs had to be considered. I also became aware that I was aggravating the patients' problems by attempting to impose my control over them.

After a year or two of my avoidance of dealing with the patients' weight issues, I was made aware of another approach. This journey was propelled by my understanding of my own control issues and disassociated behavior toward patients. A nondieting approach was being advocated by the lay press. My associate, Dana Armstrong, a Registered Dietitian, applied this approach to patients with nutrition-sensitive diseases. To my surprise, not only did the patient not "fall apart with dieting abandonment," but they actually did better. Numerous patients told me or wrote to me about the "truth" of this approach. Attending the national meetings of the "Association for the Health Enhancement of Large People" and my association with fellow professionals, Mary Tierney, Karen Carrier, and the authors of this book, helped accelerate my appreciation of the problem.

Diets, as we define them, are restrictions placed on the usual eating behavior for some particular goal. They can be restrictions of amount (calorie counting, "eat less") or a particular kind of food (eat less carbohydrates, no sugar or white flour, or counting fat grams). Regardless, they all fail.

Why? It appears that eating is done in the unaware state. This is illustrated by the frequent reports of patients sincerely reporting they do not eat that much food. However, in a study conducted in our clinic, 89% of patients claiming to be on a low salt diet, ate a salty food the night before their clinic visit. In another study, patients claiming to be unable to lose weight despite perfect compliance on our 1000 calorie liquid diet, lost 10 pounds in a controlled environment for one week with no access to other foods. Eating therefore does not seem to be any more controlled by the conscious state than breathing. Certainly we can control a breath, but for the rest of the day?

What then controls weight? Certainly genetics do. Nearly 80% of identical twins raised in separate households develop adiposity to the same level. Height and intelligence are similarly related to inheritance. How genetics influence eating is not known but one way may be heightening awareness of foods present in the environment.

Food availability also controls food consumption. An example is a clean plate. How did the server of that plate know how much food would meet that consumer's appetite? Restriction of availability, as with dieting, not only restricts another factor in controlling eating, emotional calming, but also sets up a powerful eating stimulus, deprivation. Deprivation will eventually lead to bingeing and diet failure. Thus, eating for emotional calming and for decreasing the sense of food deprivation, I feel, are the powerful stimuli for excessive eating.

The approach we use with our patients with diabetes, hypertension and hyperlipidemias incorporates acceptance of size and disease, avoidance of dieting, reduction of real and perceived deprivation by having food in abundance, increasing self-awareness by sensing hunger and the blood sugar (if a diabetic), and allowing the patient to make health choices.

How can I change the mind of my fellow health professional? We have found patients' letters to health professionals to be effective. We also like having patients referred to us who are other professionals' "worst cases" in controlling their eating. Our successes have created a grudging acceptance by some fellow physicians.

Finally, I strongly urge readers to make office settings size friendly by having large gowns, armless chairs, large blood pressure cuffs and extra wide exam tables available. Evaluate your need to weigh the patient. Don't if you do not need the information. If you do, explain to the patients why you need their weight and then weigh them in kilograms or backwards on the scale so they cannot see their weight.

Most important is how a patient feels and whether we can improve the patient outcome with this approach, and we do!

Allen King, MD, FACP
King Medical Group
Salinas, California

Introduction

Moving Away From Diets is a step by step guide to help implement a gentle, trusting counseling approach to weight, fitness and eating *without* dieting. The approach is not just for burned out dieters. We have used these components for more than ten years with clients of all ages with eating disorders, diabetes, and normal weight individuals who needed to relearn how to eat. This guide is designed for anyone who works with individuals or groups on food, eating, weight management, or self-esteem issues. You will find it especially useful if you are a health care provider (e.g. dietitian, health educator, counselor, nurse, physician, physical therapist, or exercise physiologist). Parts will be of interest to fitness instructors, wellness directors, program administrators, and educators.

The nondiet, internally regulated, "connected" approach to eating and exercise outlined here is an *alternative* to traditional weight control methods that emphasize weight loss by just eating less and exercising more. This information is essential if you seek to promote optimal nutrition, health, and well-being to people of *all* sizes, shapes, and weights.

We do not advocate a single, specific nondiet "program." No one program is the answer to every client's food and weight concerns. In fact, within the nondiet paradigm there are many variations and several different points of view. *Moving Away From Diets* will share a general framework of nondiet weight, hunger, and fitness management. It will suggest a wide variety of techniques, resources, and materials to help implement this approach. Using these strategies, you can develop your own personal nondiet "style" within the context of your practice and community.

Moving Away From The Dieting Mentality
This guide will challenge many tenets of the current diet mentality, including the beliefs that:
- it is impossible to be fit <u>and</u> fat at the same time;
- <u>all</u> large people <u>must</u> lose weight in order to improve their health and fitness level;
- all large people are in poor health;
- everyone can lose weight <u>if</u> they just follow the proper diet and regular exercise program; and,
- the main reason people regain lost weight is <u>their</u> failure to comply with prescribed diets or make long-term commitments to weight loss.

The Nondiet Challenge
Moving Away From Diets gives you a new approach to weight management and new ways to help your clients optimize their health and well-being. This guide can:
- help you move away from the frustration of prescribing restrictive diets or trying to help clients on restrictive diet regimens, and begin to experience greater satisfaction in your work;
- help clients enhance their health status and fitness level as they give up crazy diets, compulsive exercise, and body hate;
- assist you in designing programs and collaborative efforts with like-minded professionals on the cutting edge of health care;

- provide support for using a nondiet approach to build your business and enhance your practice.

We will point you in new directions, but we certainly will not provide all the answers. As the twentieth century ends, the nondiet approach is definitely a "work in progress," sometimes generating more questions than it answers. This guide is not a definitive text, but rather a starting place for your exploration into a new paradigm. Shopenhauer, the noted 19th century German philosopher, suggested that all truth passes through three stages. First it is ridiculed, then violently opposed, and finally accepted as self-evident. The nondiet movement is still being ridiculed by some and is definitely opposed by many in the diet and health care industries. It is our hope that your work with these concepts will help move the nondiet approach into the self-evident stage.

Moving Away From Diets covers the nondiet concepts in detail. In chapter 2 we discuss the critical importance of size acceptance by both providers and consumers of health care. We outline the steps you take to facilitate your clients' path to self-care. Chapters 3 discusses how the dieting cycle contributes to a person's eating problems. The three facets of HungerWork are covered in Chapters 4, 5 and 6. This treatment approach helps clients get in touch with natural signals of hunger, appetite, fullness, and satiety through identifying and decoding eating experiences to promote joyful and healthful eating. A person's body size does not determine his or her need for HungerWork. Chapter 7 covers the origins and treatment strategies for exercise resistance. Chapters 8 and 9 pull the discussion together with counseling and implementation strategies along with case studies. The final Chapter 10 discusses marketing the nondiet approach.

This book includes counseling techniques, educational materials, and a list of dozens of nondiet resources. Before discussing the details, it covers several fundamental issues, including terminology, outcomes, evaluation, and scope of practice.

Along with this book, we have camera-ready handouts and self-study courses available that will help you better understand and implement the nondiet approach.

Closing...

Dayle Hayes, MS, RD, LD
Nancy King, MS, RD, CDE
Karen Kratina, MA, RD, LD

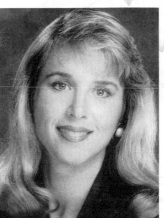

KARIN KRATINA, MA, RD, a Nutrition Therapist and exercise physiologist, is pursuing a PhD in Psychological Anthropology at the University of Florida focusing on woman's relationship with food, eating, and weight in this culture. In 1990, she developed and directed nutrition and exercise services at The Renfrew Center of Coconut Creek, Florida, a residential facility specializing in the treatment of women with eating disorders and other mental health concerns. She now serves there as a Training Consultant. She has worked as a sports nutritionist for the Lady Gators at UF and currently is in private practice in Gainesville, Florida.

Ms. Kratina regularly presents at national and international, and is published and frequently quoted in professional journals as well as the popular press. She is Disordered Eating Editor for the SCAN's (Sports and Cardiovascular Nutritionists) newsletter, *PULSE,* and a regular contributor to the National Eating Disorders Organization's (NEDO) newsletter. Her publications include "Treatment of Eating Disorders" in *Handbook of Medical Nutrition Therapy: The Florida Diet Manual* (1995,1999), "Nutrition Education and Therapy" in The Eating Disorder SourceBook, and "Exercise Recommendations, Resistance and Compulsion" in *Nutrition Therapy: Advanced Counseling Skills* (1995).

ACKNOWLEDGMENTS: My passion for this work is nurtured by my mother, Sandra H. Kratina, PhD, whose acceptance of my ideas even when she doesn't quite understand them, made this book possible. Additionally, she and my friend, Elinor Robin, have been my ever faithful editors. Although neither were able to edit this book, their assistance has been invaluable to me throughout my career.

I want to acknowledge Sister Waldia Warden, who believed in me; Carl Davis, whose support and passion for my work has been invaluable; Adrienne Ressler, the expert; and The Renfrew Center where so many of my ideas were and continue to be, solidified. Thanks also to my clients from whom I continue to receive direction in my work; and last but not least, to my co-authors, both incredibly brilliant women from whom I have learned a great deal.

E-mail: KKratina@aol.com

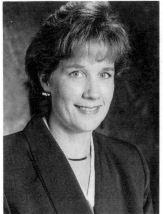

Nancy L. King, MS, RD, CDE is a registered dietitian, certified diabetes educator, and exercise physiologist residing in Southern California. In 1987 Nancy founded Nutrition Designs, a nutrition counseling center specializing in a nondiet approach to disordered eating, diabetes, and personal wellness. She assists individuals in breaking away from restrictive diets and nutrition regimens that can create both disordered eating and exercise patterns, and guides them in learning self-acceptance and self-regulation of food, weight, and movement.

Ms. King is a recognized speaker both locally and nationally. Recent presentations include: American Dietetic Association annual meetings in Orlando 1994 and Chicago 1995, as well as the 1996 California Dietetic Association annual meeting, and the Los Angeles Dietetic Association in 1995. Ms. King promotes pleasurable eating and movement through her writing and is published in several journals, including *On the Cutting Edge,* SCAN's *PULSE,* and *The Healthy Weight Journal.*

STATEMENT: As I look around at the wonder of nature, I appreciate the shady oak tree for its strength to hold a tire swing, the weeping willow for its gracefulness, the great California redwoods for their majesty, and the maple tree for its exquisite autumn color parade. Likewise, beautiful, healthy bodies come in all shapes, sizes and colors with countless unique abilities and cherished differences.

Shortly after starting my private practice, I recognized diets didn't translate well from "paper" to real life. Through listening to my clients share their experiences of modifying their eating and exercise behavior through dieting, one common thread is hunger. They are hungry... and they experience hunger as a problem. Many clients do not know what they hunger for, but they know it isn't restrained eating and compulsory exercise. They hunger for peace and health through eating, joy and vitality through movement, and love and growth through self-acceptance. *Moving Away From Diets* serves as a map to guide individuals on their journey to satisfying their hunger and embracing themselves.

x

ACKNOWLEDGMENTS: I thank my clients for sharing their lives with me. They are a source of inspiration and growth; being a part of their journey is an honor. I am grateful to Karin Kratina for her wisdom and leadership, as well as her ingenuity and passion for this work. I thank Dayle Hayes for sharing her gift of artistry through words. Fortunately, we are never truly done! Kathy King Helm, our publisher, has been instrumental in this project as she has reminded me of the "forest while I was amidst the trees." And, I have been blessed daily by my devoted office manager, sane-maker, Leslie Modes. Through her graceful spirit and zeal for my work, she supports and encourages me to stretch beyond my limits.

I cherish the profound observation our son Jeffrey made at 7 years old, "Getting thin really doesn't help you, because then you can't stand up. That's why Barbie can't stand up." And I appreciate the simple response Andy, our six year old gave when I asked him how he knows when to eat, "I know I need to eat when my stomach feels wobbly. I stop when the wobbly's gone." I wonder why it would ever need to be more complicated than that? I am deeply grateful to Tom King, my life partner and trusted advisor. His belief in me and shared passion for my work keeps me focused, driven, and balanced (at least in pursuit of the latter.) Finally, I thank God for creating us as individuals; unique and diverse.

For information on HungerWork Seminars   call: (818) 957-8588 or (818) 790-8588 or E-mail: NancyLKing@aol.com

Dayle Hayes MS, RD, LD is a nutrition consultant, speaker, and author whose creative approach to healthful eating has attracted national recognition. Early in her career, Dayle realized that diets did not work. Since then, she 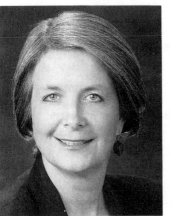 has developed many innovative programs to teach the benefits of nutrition without dieting. Her video, BODY TRUST: Undieting Your Weigh to Health and Happiness, received a Bronze WorldFest Award at the 1994 Houston International Film and Video Festival.

Dayle works extensively with the media in Montana and nationally. She has been quoted in *USA Today, The New York Times, The Chicago Tribune, Cooking Light, Ladies Home Journal, McCall's, Family Circle, Prevention, Runner's World,* and *Working Mother.* She authored Put Your Best Food Forward, created the nutrition game, 5 a Day BINGO, and produced two other videos: Beans, Peas, and Broccoli Trees and Getting a Head Start with 5 a Day.

In 1994 Dayle was elected to the board of directors of the American Dietetic Association, where she serves as co-chair of the ADA Technology Task Force. In recognition of her creativity and dedication, she has received numerous local and national honors, including a Consulting Nutritionist Leadership Award (1990); Montana Dietitian of the Year (1991); an Excellence in Nutrition Education Award (1991); the first Anita Owen Award for Innovative Nutrition Education Programs for the Public (1991); a Governor's Health Promotion Award (1992); a Centers for Disease Control and Prevention Outstanding Community Health Promotion Program Award (1993); a Montana Advertising Federation Addy Award (1994), and a Head Start Program Outstanding Community Service Award (1995).

STATEMENT: In graduate school I was trained to put people on diets. When I began to practice nutrition in the real world, it became clear, almost immediately, that most diets fail. Now, after almost two decades as a practicing nutritionist, I have come to believe that there are only three things that people can do to manage their weight: learn to feed their body healthfully, move their body joyfully, and love their body unconditionally.

I readily admit that size acceptance--learning to love and care for the body you have--is not an easy task. Any kind of self-acceptance is extraordinarily hard in our fat phobic, diet obsessed world. I am incredibly impressed by anyone, especially large women, who have done the hard work necessary to stop hating their bodies and themselves.

Size acceptance is difficult, but not impossible. Fortunately, there are many ways you can help your clients along the path. And, I believe that it is worth every ounce of effort that we put into it, as individuals, as professionals, and as a society.

ACKNOWLEDGMENTS: My work on the Body Trust concepts has been possible because of my clients. Their willingness to share their struggles and their triumphs has enabled me to expand my views of nutrition, health, and weight. I am grateful for their trust and for the opportunity to challenge old beliefs and discover new frontiers.

I am ever grateful to my family for their love and support. It is their trust that makes my explorations possible.

Body Trust phone: (800) 321-9499 E-mail: EatRightMT@aol.com

1

The Big Picture

[You] could be the first to break the equation linking body weight to moral or psychological status, to judge clients and neighbors for who they are and not for what they weigh, to examine [your] own attitudes toward people who are overweight, and to work to overcome negative stereotypes (1).

THE BOTTOM LINE: DO DIETS DO MORE HARM THAN GOOD?
Interventions based on shame, blame, and starvation have failed to stem, and may be contributing, to the increased prevalence of obesity in the United States (2).

Moving Away From Diets challenges you to question the current diet paradigm and consider adopting the nondiet paradigm. The most compelling reason to move from traditional diets to the nondiet approach is, quite simply, that most diets fail. This failure is certainly no secret. You know it, we know it, obesity researchers know it, every faithful dieter knows it, and it is broadcast on the cover of magazines from *Time* to *People*.

Our nation spends over $30 billion a year on dieting (3). According to a 1996 survey by the Calorie Control Council, about 46 million people in the U.S. (24% percent of the population) are on a diet (4). For decades Americans have been popping diet pills, drinking diet soda, reading diet books, and joining diet programs in droves. At the same time, we have been getting fatter and fatter. Despite the efforts of a gigantic diet industry, thousands of health care professionals, and dozens of dedicated scientists, "(no) one has yet found a satisfactory way to achieve long-term weight reduction that works on a population-wide basis (5)."

It is true that many people lose weight by dieting, and that a select few are able to maintain their loss over time. However, it is well documented that most weight loss is not sustained (6). The oft-quoted statistics are that in 95% of cases, lost weight is regained within five years, and that a consistent minority of dieters gain back more weight than they lose (7). Even the staunchest diet defenders concede that "[Research shows] poor long-term results from clinical treatment trials on obesity and most individuals return to baseline (8)."

Although the diet debate will undoubtedly rage for years to come it is clear that with current treatments, permanent weight loss is not possible for an overwhelming majority of people. As health providers, we must confront what is essentially a question of values. If most diets do not result in sustainable weight loss, is it advisable or ethical to continue to promote and prescribe them for everyone? *The bottom line is: do diets do more harm than good?*

Like numerous other health care professionals (1,2,9), we have examined the evidence and come to a decisive conclusion. *For us, the downside of dieting outweighs the temporary benefits of weight loss seen in many weight management programs.* The problems with the diet culture in the U.S., acknowledged by researchers on both sides of the diet debate include (8,9):

- concerns about the physical and psychological impact of the pressure to continuously diet, especially for women;
- risks of increasing the incidence of eating disorders given the cultural context of beauty (for example: gaunt images of role models);
- changes in the relationship between chronic dieters and the food they eat, including an increased preference for high-fat, high-sugar foods;
- increases in the tendency to overeat or binge seen in restrained eaters and chronic dieters;
- questions regarding the psychological impact of blaming individuals for their weight status or diet failure;
- effects of discrimination against fat children in schools and fat adults at work;
- disturbing data on the long-term health consequences of certain weight reduction methods, and weight loss and thinness in general.

The Council on Size and Weight Discrimination summarized these points in their *"Top Ten Reasons To Give Up Dieting"* (10) flyer, which is useful for group discussions and talking with the media, see Figure 1-A.

Traditional Weight Control Model

Despite concerns about diet failure rates, the traditional weight control model argues that diets are necessary because obesity is a chronic, degenerative, life-threatening "illness" (6,8). According to this model, people with obesity must diet to reach and maintain a recommended body weight in order to be healthy.

The traditional medical model teaches there is a lean optimal body weight for all persons, and that the incidence of disease and premature death increases in direct proportion to body weight. This is *not* true for all heavy individuals. If this were the case, the majority of heavy individuals would have adult onset diabetes and most heavy women would get breast cancer. ***Whether obesity is an actual health risk, and to what extent, varies substantially between individuals (11,12). It must be pointed out that definite health risks also can result from some methods of weight loss, and with weight cycling (yo-yo dieting) in some chronic dieters (7,13,14).*** Some researchers are also beginning to raise questions about the restrictiveness of the current government weight guidelines (15,16).

A nondiet approach may seem a radical departure, in reality, it is quite conservative. For example, medical procedures, medications and programs are required to be both <u>safe</u> and <u>effective</u>. Practitioners, institutions, and government agencies like the Food and Drug Administration (FDA) use standards of safety and efficacy to evaluate new proposals. When applying these standards to the current spectrum of weight loss methods, the answer is straight forward. ***Many diets and weight loss gimmicks are not safe, and few are effective in the long run.***

We, like a growing number of health and fitness professionals, believe that new approaches and new definitions of weight control success are necessary because the current paradigm "is scientifically invalid, inappropriate from a behavioral perspective, and ethically unacceptable (2)."

Fortunately, making the shift to the nondiet approach is not as difficult as it might seem. Nondiet messages are based on common sense and supported by increasing scientific evidence. The basic concepts are simple and positive. (See The Nondiet Approach, Figure 1-B.) They can make a powerful impact on personal and public health, and therefore on the well-being of individuals and of nations.

World Wide Movement

In some countries, even the government recognizes the potential health benefits and cost savings of nondiet programs. For example, the Canadian office of health promotion has introduced an innovative

Figure 1-A

Top Ten Reasons To Give Up Dieting

#10: Diets don't work. Even if you lose weight, you will probably gain it all back and you might gain back more than you lost.

#9: Diets are expensive. If you did not buy special diet products, you could save enough to get new clothes, which would improve your outlook right now.

#8: Diets are boring. People on diets talk and think about food and practically nothing else. There's a lot more to life.

#7: Diets don't necessarily improve your health. Like the weight loss, health improvement is temporary. Dieting can actually cause health problems.

#6: Diets don't make you beautiful. Very few people will ever look like models. Glamour is a look, not a size. You don't have to be thin to be attractive.

#5: Diets are not sexy. If you want to feel and be more attractive, take care of your body and your appearance. Feeling healthy makes you look your best.

#4: Diets can turn into eating disorders. The obsession to be thin can lead to anorexia, bulimia, bingeing, and compulsive exercising.

#3: Diets can make you afraid of food. Food nourishes and comforts us, and gives us pleasure. Dieting can make food seem like your enemy, and can deprive you of all the positive things about food.

#2: Diets can rob you of energy. If you want to lead a full and active life, you need good nutrition, and enough food to meet your body's needs.

#1: Learning to love and accept yourself just as you are will give you self-confidence, better health, and a sense of well-being that will last a lifetime.

program called *"Vitality"* to the entire country (17). This integrated effort shifts the focus away from weight loss and nutrient avoidance, and takes a fresh approach to promoting nutrition and physical fitness.

Vitality, along with its public and private partners (e.g. health providers, worksite wellness programs, the media, and the food, fitness, and fashion industries), is dedicated to promoting three positive ideas:

- Take pleasure in eating a variety of foods by listening to internal hunger cues.
- Enjoy a range of moderate, fun physical activities as part of a daily routine.
- Accept and recognize that healthy bodies come in a range of weights, shapes, and sizes.

NEW MEASUREMENTS: How do we determine success?

Good health is more than a number on a scale. It's waking up feeling good. It's having energy. It's knowing you can depend on your body to do the things you want to do (18).

One of the first questions that professionals ask about a nondiet approach is, "does it work?" Some skeptics would say there is a lack of scientific evidence for the success of any nondiet program. To be perfectly honest, that was true. However, there is growing evidence today. Success is measured in terms of improved eating, fitness, clinical assessments and mental health, not simply the measurement of the past: absolute weight loss and return to the chart "ideal" weight.

The nondiet paradigm is still in its infancy, thus the results of research and program evaluations are just beginning to be published (see studies below). Funding is often a limiting factor in research; there is no current funding for large scale, long-term evaluations of nondiet work. Research money is short in part because no industry stands to benefit financially from supporting such research. Government grants tend to support more traditional medical models of weight loss by diet and exercise, although the National Institutes of Health has begun to consider evaluation of nondiet programs.

Ethical beliefs may also limit research on the effects of the new paradigm on weight parameters. Some practitioners make a conscious choice *not* to weigh their program participants, believing that weight preoccupation is a significant part of the problem with diet failure and overeating. The more subjective measures of success they do report may not be as acceptable to some scientists and journals. In fact, some nondiet advocates (19) report substantial resistance to the publication of their work, a not uncommon phenomenon when a new approach challenges the well entrenched status quo.

Research and program evaluation can be expensive and tedious tasks but they are essential to accurately assess the impact of the nondiet approach and convince others of its validity. We agree that rigorous scientific review of this new approach is necessary. We also recognize that just as new paradigms require new terminology, they may also require new methods for measuring outcomes.

We urge practitioners of this approach to familiarize themselves with the existing research and to implement an evaluation component in their programs. It is essential to measure outcomes with:

- standard medical data (e.g. glucose, blood lipids, and blood pressure);
- assessment of food intake and eating behaviors;
- fitness parameters such as oxygen uptake (VO_2 max), strength and flexibility;
- more subjective analyses, like those mentioned below in the *Handbook* (20).

The question of whether to use weight measurement is up to the practitioner and the setting of the program. Some would argue weight should never be measured, while others suggest using it as one criterion among many.

The Handbook of Assessment Methods for Eating Behaviors and Weight Related Problems (20) provides reliable tests, tools, and questionnaires for evaluation purposes. This volume, edited by a National Institutes of Health (NIH) obesity researcher, includes a variety of instruments you can use with individuals and groups to assess the effects of a nondiet approach. Some useful tools included in this volume are the *Satisfaction with Life Scale; Rosenberg Self-esteem Scale; Beliefs about Obese Persons*

Scale; *Minnesota Satisfaction Questionnaire*; *Attitudes about Weight and Dieting*; *Fat Phobia Scale*; and *Forbidden Food Survey*.

Nondiet Research Results

In published research, Ciliska (21) studied the effects of a 12-week group session (both educational and experiential) on "chronically obese women." She reported improvements in self-esteem, restrained eating and bulimia, and short term improvements in body dissatisfaction, drive for thinness, depression, and social adjustment. Weight, percentage average weight, blood pressure, fasting glucose, serum cholesterol, and lipids were unchanged by the intervention and at 6-month posttest.

Carrier, et al. (22) reported significant improvements over three years in various assessments of self-esteem, self-acceptance, self-nourishment, and restrained eating. Their worksite wellness program also reported an increase in level of physical activity. Although the researchers chose not to measure body weight, they recommend that future studies include physiological measures. Polivy and Herman (23) reported similar results in a 6-month follow-up of a 10-week "undieting" group.

Omichinski and Harrison (24) used pre- and post-quizzes to analyze the effects of a 10-week nondiet group in Canada, and reported significant improvement in self-acceptance and self-nourishment scales. The authors acknowledge the limitations of the self-reported data and the lack of more objective data such as food diaries or physiological measures. A similar Australian program using 10-week groups did report a mean weight loss of 3.1 kg at 2-year follow-up (25). A nondiet approach to diabetes management by Armstrong and King (26), has shown changes in both objective measures (improvements in blood glucose control and gradual weight loss that is maintained over time) and more subjective measures (feelings of control and self-esteem; modification of compulsive and restrained eating; and reduction in guilt).

Steinhardt and Nagel (27) evaluated the effects of a nondiet program on the problem of compulsive overeating in a sample of readers of *Overcoming Overeating*. While acknowledging the limitations of their convenience sample and the lack of physiological measures, they report decreases in eating preoccupation, body preoccupation, and emotional overeating over a 2-year period, particularly for individuals who implemented the mechanics of the curriculum.

NEW DIRECTIONS: WHAT IS A NONDIET APPROACH?

We must intervene without making the situation worse. To this end, (we wish) to see, instead of a group of diet victims, a population of varied sizes, in good physical and mental health (28).

Using a nondiet approach is a new way of life for some health care providers. For others, it is a natural progression toward a gentler, more accepting model of health care. It does mean challenging what many of us learned in school and training programs, and taking a closer look at our beliefs, assumptions, and professional practices. It may also mean making fundamental changes in the "usual" relationship between providers and consumers of health services.

We want to make one point clear: the nondiet approach is *not* an "anti-health" model. Some critics of the nondiet movement seem to believe that recognizing the failure of restrictive diets means encouraging people to forget nutrition and health altogether. Nothing could be further from the truth.

Moving away from diets means focusing on *total* health rather than on the number of pounds on the scale. This holistic, nondiet view recognizes the many dimensions of personal health, including its physical, emotional, mental, and spiritual aspects. Weight is only a single measurement, which may or may not have a direct bearing on health status. ***Being overweight according to the height and weight charts does not automatically imply poor health, just as being "ideal weight" does not guarantee good health.*** In the nondiet approach, the overall goal is to support a healthy lifestyle, by focusing on four basic tenets, Figure 1-B.

Figure 1-B
The Nondiet Approach

1. Total health enhancement and well-being, rather than weight loss or achieving a specific "ideal weight."
2. Self-acceptance and respect for the diversity of healthy, beautiful bodies, rather than the pursuit of an idealized weight at all cost.
3. The pleasure of eating well, based on internal cues of hunger and satiety, rather than on external food plans or diets.
4. The joy of movement, encouraging all physical activities rather than prescribing a specific routine of regimented exercise.

Moving Away From Diets covers each of these four concepts in detail. Before discussing the details, it covers several fundamental issues, including terminology, outcomes, evaluation, and scope of practice. Figure 1-C, Weight Management: Traditional vs. The Nondiet Approach, on the next page contrasts the traditional diet paradigm with the nondiet approach.

NEW WORDS: HOW DO WE SAY WHAT WE MEAN?
Paradigms are the theoretical frameworks by which professional practices are formulated, evaluated, and adapted. Successfully shifting from one paradigm to another often requires a shift in terminology, because the "usual" words and phrases can keep us stuck in old ways of thinking. Whether written or spoken, words have a powerful effect on how people perceive and react to messages. The words used in the weight arena are particularly emotional and value-laden, especially for large people and restrained eaters.

If you want to communicate a message effectively, you have to choose your words carefully. Consider how precisely a public relations agency selects words for an advertising campaign. They know exactly the audience reaction they want and they pick their words accordingly. The terminology you choose for verbal communications and written materials is equally important, especially for a new approach.

"DIET" First, consider the word *diet*. Many Americans quickly identify it as a four-letter word, and even Richard Simmons notes that the first three letters spell die! Ask any audience their reaction to "diet." You will hear a chorus of negative words like deprivation, restrictive, hungry, rigid, boring, starvation, limited, regimented, abstinence, or no chocolate!

The dictionary provides several definitions. Most professionals would be comfortable with Webster's first definition: "food and drink regularly provided or consumed" or "habitual nourishment." However, anyone who has dieted might closely identify with "to cause to eat and drink sparingly or according to prescribed rules (29)."

Fortunately, there are several, more positive terms to use in place of diet. The exact one that you choose will depend on your audience and your message. Consider the following alternatives, and your reaction to them:

- eating style or eating pattern
- fuel, nourishment
- food intake or food you eat
- joyful eating, pleasurable eating
- physically-connected eating
- internally regulated, nonrestrained eating

Table 1-C

Weight Management: Traditional vs. The Nondiet Approach

	Diet Paradigm	Nondiet Approach
WEIGHT	Achieving and maintaining ideal weight as close as possible, used as measure of success.	Body will seek its natural weight as individual eats in response to physical cues of hunger and fullness, as well as a sense of well-being and pleasure.
HUNGER	Attempt to suppress or ignore hunger. Transgressions associated with lack of will power or "giving in." Physical and emotional hunger confused.	Physical cues to eat are valued and relied upon. Responding to physical hunger and fullness (with occasional emotional eating) will bring about natural weight.
EXERCISE	Reaching and maintaining goal weight is dependent on exercise, which is often dropped when individual falls off diet. It is seen as a "have to" or "should," which commonly produces exercise resistance.	Physical activity, listening to body, seeking play, and natural movement are explored. Not connected to weight loss or change of body size or shape.
FOOD	Moralized as good/bad, legal/ illegal, should/shouldn't, on/off diet. Variety, quantity, calories, fat grams, etc., determined by external source, i. e. the diet, health care provider, the parent, etc.	Neutralized. All food is acceptable. Quantity, quality, and frequency are determined by individual exploring and responding to physical cues, sense of well-being, taste, and medical values (such as blood glucose levels). It is self-regulated, internally cued, and nonrestrained.
SELF-ESTEEM and SIZE ACCEPTANCE	Individual typically gains a false sense of power and control with weight loss, adherence to diet, and exercise plan. Self-esteem and body acceptance rarely improve. This goal is elusive as one can get thinner, more toned, or both.	Increase in self-esteem and personal power from self-determined eating style and movement. Bodies come in all sizes and are naturally beautiful. Cultural norms are recognized as hazardous; pursuit of these standards can interfere with quality of life.
TRUST/ DISTRUST of SELF and BODY	Individual may come to distrust body and sense of judgment, especially with history of failure. Trust is placed primarily in diet or provider.	Trust develops in self and body by discerning physical cues and freely responding to them without judgment or criticism.

"FOOD" Some health providers tend to describe food in clinical terms. It is natural, especially for dietitians, to talk about nutrients, proteins, amino acids, saturated fats, and phytochemicals. Unfortunately, in the midst of our scientific jargon, we sometimes forget that the number one reason why people choose food is *taste!*

One goal of the nondiet approach is to move away from the dichotomy of good food versus bad food. In our work we promote the joy of eating well, and focus on the pleasurable aspects of food rather than on the avoidance of certain nutrients. This means integrating the science of nutrition with the art of preparing and consuming tasteful food.

One of the best ways to inspire others to *enjoy* the benefits of healthful eating is to use the language of great chefs and successful cooks. As practically any cookbook will demonstrate, food lovers discuss the taste, aromas, colors, textures, and the myriad flavors of their products. When you talk about food and nutrition, use words and phrases like:

- delicious, flavorful, or tasty
- pungent, delicate, or robust
- lemon-yellow, bright-orange, or emerald-green
- crunchy, smooth, or creamy
- spicy, sweet, or sublime

"EXERCISE" This is another word that can easily get in the way of pleasure. Even though the dictionary defines exercise as "bodily exertion for the sake of developing or maintaining physical fitness" (29), the typical reaction may be considerably more negative and much less pleasurable. Exercise is often synonymous with images of a sweaty, painful workout!

Getting people in the U.S. off their couches and onto the streets requires a more positive and creative approach. Rather than tell you exactly what terms to use, we have provided a list of some alternative words that may be appropriate, depending on your style, your audience, and your situation. Think about the effect of substituting one of the following terms for exercise:

- play
- joyful movement
- physical activity
- active lifestyle
- vitality

"SIZE" The words used to describe *size* are especially critical. Although commonly used in clinical settings, many large people are offended by the terms *"obese"* and *"overweight."* Both feel harsh and judgmental to some and imply a comparison to an ideal status to others. ("You can't possibly be healthy, because you are an obese female.")

Fat is an even more complicated word. For many, it brings back the memories of childhood taunts like "fatso" or "fatty." The implication of "fat" for them is intensely negative--as in fat is bad and thin is good. On the other hand, some activists in the size acceptance movement consciously use the word "fat" in order to neutralize the term and reclaim it in a more positive sense.

The exact words you choose to describe large people will depend upon your setting and audience. The important part of the process is defining and challenging the existing stereotypes implied in various words. You may want to consider using:

- large-sized
- endowed
- full-figured
- big

- abundant
- ample
- graced

Here are just a few of the other terms that you may want to consider as you speak or write about the nondiet approach:

Old words: *healthy food or healthy behavior*
New words: health enhancing nourishing fueling

Old words: *prescribe, treat, instruct, or teach*
New words: guide counsel motivate
empower educate inspire
listen validate

Old words: *should eat or must avoid*
New words: select choose enjoy
discover experiment explore

Old words: *weight control, weight management,* or *weight loss*
New words: fitness healthy living joyful living

Positive Terminology is Becoming More Popular

Many other words, phrases, and descriptors have negative and judgmental connotations, especially to longtime dieters and large people. Using them can get in the way of your message and the success of your program. You may want to change, or at least evaluate them, as you begin to use a nondiet approach.

As an example of positive terminology in action, the Dietary Guidelines Alliance used focus groups to develop messages which consumers found personally motivating, attainable, and realistic (30). The Alliance, a partnership of U.S. health organizations, government agencies, and food producer groups, built its entire theme on the cornerstone of enjoyment-- of food, taste, and physical activity.

The Alliance theme (**"It's All About You"**) is one example of using a nondiet approach in public education programs. Their materials suggest that individuals "make healthy choices that fit your lifestyle so you can do the things you want to do." The key messages of the campaign are (30):

Be Realistic: Make small changes over time in what you eat and the level of activity you do. After all, small steps work better than giant leaps.

Be Adventurous: Expand your tastes to enjoy a variety of foods.

Be Flexible: Go ahead and balance what you eat and the physical activity you do over several days. No need to worry about just one day or one meal.

Be Sensible: Enjoy all food, just don't overdo it.

Be Active: Walk the dog, don't just watch the dog walk.

WORDS OF WISDOM: IS A NONDIET APPROACH APPROPRIATE FOR EVERYONE?
The goal for all should be a healthful lifestyle that can be maintained indefinitely, rather than a short term "diet" that will most likely be abandoned and produce more overweight and psychological discomfort (31).

We believe some aspects of a nondiet approach can benefit anyone. For example, the unconditional acceptance and nurturing terminology of this new paradigm are appropriate for all clients, whatever their medical status or diagnosis. We also recognize a nondiet approach will be more successful for some individuals than others. Chapter 6 discusses the issue of when to use aggressive medical nutrition therapy versus a nondiet approach.

This new paradigm is especially useful for clients of any weight with a history of yo-yo dieting (repeated episodes of weight loss and regain). Unfortunately, health care professionals most often single out large people, especially women and very heavy men, for strict weight reduction diets without considering their past dieting history. This group often responds to a new approach that focuses on healing eating problems and exercise resistance.

In our experience, the clients who benefit most from an intensive nondiet approach are those who:

- have made repeated unsuccessful attempts to diet, follow restrictive nutrition plans, change their eating patterns, or lose weight;
- feel uncomfortable or fearful around food;
- are out of touch with hunger, fullness, appetite, and satiety cues;
- eat compulsively, binge eat, or restrict food;
- experience food as unsatisfying most of the time;
- start and drop exercise, resist an active lifestyle, or exercise compulsively;
- connect their self-esteem and self-worth with their weight, food intake, exercise, or appearance;
- assume their total health hinges upon degree of control over their nutrition-sensitive disease (i.e. diabetes or hypertension).

In addition, the individuals best suited for this approach are:

- basically healthy (although they may have a chronic disease, such as diabetes, hypertension, or arthritis or physical limitations);
- able to invest time and energy in a process-oriented approach to change (as opposed to a more didactic program);
- able to do nondiet work on an individual basis, in free or low cost support groups, or they have the financial resources (personal or insurance) to attend sessions and group meetings as necessary.

Using the Nondiet Approach with Children, Teens and Adults

The nondiet concepts can be used successfully with people of any age, including children and teens. There is general agreement that strict weight reduction diets are unsuitable for most young people because they can compromise growth and may lead to disordered eating patterns (32). Many experts recommend youth programs that focus on lifestyle changes and positive body image without restrictive diets (33,34). There are also specific nondiet programs and resources designed for both children (34,35) and teens (33,36).

As with the development of any treatment plan, the initial assessment for a nondiet approach includes a review of the client's physical and mental health status. Any paradigm of care, including a nondiet approach, will encounter barriers to improved health in some individuals. Some clients have a poor prognosis with any approach due to:

- critical, progressive, or terminal illness,
- dual or multiple diagnoses such as severe depression or other mental illness,
- late intervention,
- relationship crises,
- difficulties in comprehension;
- financial limitations,
- infrequent contact with the health care system.

PUTTING IT INTO PRACTICE: WILL NONDIET WORK IN YOUR SETTING?

This approach can work in any type of setting from public health and education to acute care and outpatient clinics. Whatever the setting, you may want to consider some questions before deciding to implement a nondiet approach:

- Are you and your staff completely committed to moving away from diets when it is appropriate for an individual or group?
- Do you provide a "size friendly" atmosphere for your clients and customers? (See Chapter 2.)
- Do you know the limits of your particular type of practice and involve other appropriate professionals in team-centered treatment?
- Do you recognize that a nondiet approach is a process that may take some time?

KEYS TO SUCCESS

Some health professionals have difficulty making a complete commitment to a nondiet approach. Although they acknowledge that diets often don't work, they still prescribe some version of "eat less and exercise more." To successfully implement this approach, you have to believe the concept will work and not confuse clients with mixed messages. Diet "double speak" can lead to treatment dropouts and exacerbate clients' physical and psychological problems (37).

Another key to the successful implementation of a nondiet approach is to know the limits of your own practice. In other words, know the limits of your own expertise (and perhaps the limits of your state license), and know when it is appropriate to refer a client to someone else. It is best to have a complete list of local health providers, counselors, fitness professionals, and image consultants who are size friendly and who use an approach that is similar to yours. That way you can help your clients get the complete, and nonbiased health care they deserve.

Weight, eating, self-image, and food issues are at the central core of our beings. Because many large people have been victims of size discrimination, and thus internalized abuse, they may suffer from low self-esteem, social isolation, passivity, and self-hatred (38). Years of dieting may have depleted their nutritional status, destroyed their normal relationship with food, or both (11). Large people may also avoid seeking the health care they need due to embarrassment or the desire to avoid harassment (39). Unfortunately, for a large person, health care providers often lead the list of unaccepting, judgmental people they encounter.

For these reasons, chronic dieters may have multiple health needs when they finally encounter the nondiet approach. Rather than trying to take care of everything, it is vital to connect them with the gentle and concerned professionals they need in these areas of expertise:

For medical care: internist, primary care physician, or family doctor; nurse practitioner or health care center

For comprehensive nutrition services: registered dietitian, nutrition therapist (especially practitioner with outpatient counseling experience)

For fitness needs: personal trainer, fitness instructor, or physical therapist; health club or community facility; equipment distributor

For psychological counseling: mental health counselor, psychologist, or social worker; art or movement therapist; psychiatrist (if medication is necessary); support groups

For fashion needs: image consultant or personal shopper; size friendly stores and catalogs

For adaptive equipment: occupational therapist

A "team" of size friendly professionals might exist within a single facility or be spread throughout a community. However, the team develops, it is essential all members have a similar size friendly philosophy and nondiet approach. If you are not personally familiar with the work of some potential team members, use the following resource to discuss the issues with them: Figure 1-D, "Speaking Patiently" letter on pages 13 and 14.

The role of the health provider in the nondiet approach is to facilitate a path to self-care. Unlike a diet, this new paradigm is no quick fix, and promoting it takes a gentle hand and a patient personality. It might take a while for your colleagues to accept a new way of looking at weight and food issues, and it certainly takes a while for most dieters to shift gears. According to Dr. Allen King, a diabetes specialist committed to the nondiet approach, it "takes one to five years for patients to stop dieting, learn to eat what they want--and want what they know is best for their health (40)."

Figure 1-C

Speaking Patiently

I AM SURE that this letter comes as a surprise to you since I rarely make medical appointments (except when uncomfortably ill) and patients rarely write their doctors before seeing them. I am not an exceedingly resistant patient yet have unique concerns that are rarely recognized or taken seriously by health professionals.

The problem is that I have a health condition that literally overshadows and obscures the true state of my well being. While my dilemma is intensely personal, I think that the issues I raise may characterize the feelings of many of your patients facing similar circumstances. My intention is to aid you in your understanding and treatment of me as an obese person.

There is a barrier between health professionals and myself. My weight is a message from me to the doctors to keep their distance. Distance is created by the moral, social, and psychological values that prevent you and I from diagnosing my ailments and enabling me to live a more healthy life.

Here are four principles I would like to discuss with you as groundwork for working together on my health problems.

- Obesity is a medical condition, not a moral failure.
- Obese people and health professionals need to recognize the detrimental effects of yo-yo dieting.
- Obesity obscures diagnosis through generalization and shame.
- The establishment of respectful, trusting relationships with non-prejudiced doctors are of utmost importance.

1. Medical condition not a moral failure

It can be argued historically that when a health concern is not thoroughly understood and amenable to therapy, it tends to be approached from a moral perspective. The definitive example of this today is AIDS but, since that may be too explosive and close to us right now, I suggest that we think of cholera.

Cholera was painted with the brush of moralism in the early decades of this century. The health care professionals of that day observed that it was the poor who became infected. Cholera was therefore considered a result of uncleanliness, laziness and even moral degradation. When the medical view of the disease shifted as more 'hard facts" became available, the attitude and feelings about who got the disease and why altered.

Who has obesity and why are questions that are only now coming slowly into focus. With continued research chronic obesity will be better understood, controlled, and perhaps even cured. Until the research is completed, we struggle with the temptation to think of obese people in outdated, stereotypical ways--as undisciplined gluttons who willfully give in to their urges to eat. If breakthroughs are to be made, then both patients and health care consultants must break the habit of moralism. This will require the humility to say we do not have a cure for morbid obesity but while we are waiting we will not blame patients or do anything that makes the situation more unbearable than it already is for many. This is the first prerequisite for our doctor-patient partnership.

2. The detrimental effects of yo-yo dieting

Until recently, the recommended way to treat obesity was through restrictive dieting. Sometimes behavior modification and drug treatment augmented this approach. With the discovery of the yo-yo effect, there is an understandable and legitimate resistance in obese persons to any form of dieting. Obesity may contribute to a shortened life but dieting can kill you quickly. Recently there have been studies, sponsored by weight loss organizations, which suggest that yo-yo dieting is not as much a health risk as purported. Such a claim must be examined in light of the motives of these organizations who financially benefit from this form of therapy.

I have pledged to give up quick weight loss strategies because of the effects of yo-yo dieting on my health. I have lost tremendous amounts of weight through restrictive dieting, up to 175 pounds at a time. Upon completing one cycle of such dieting I had my gall bladder removed and now I have an even harder time moderating my weight than before. As if it was a great medical secret, the surgeon took me aside and told me jokingly that he called gall bladder procedures "the diet operation." Unfortunately, it was a doctor who first recommended radical weight loss. The entire experience was demoralizing.

Restriction and the so-called use of willpower do not address the problems of obese people. If *for* many, *but not all* obese patients, food is a substitute for a lack of nurturance, then the withdrawal of the food leaves the primal need for love unanswered. Restriction in diet Is not about taking control of your health but, consciously or unconsciously, will be identified with punishment and the withdrawal of comfort. The realistic statistic of 95% failure rate in permanent weight loss due to dieting does nothing to promote it as the therapy of choice for obesity.

Nevertheless, doctors, patients, and the exploitive weight loss industry collude in recommending restrictive dieting as a way of dealing with weight difficulties.

Even when this ineffective treatment is abandoned, another problem often complicates it. When a "cure" (dieting) seems hopeless, many patients experience outrage. This may take the form of indiscriminate eating. To avoid the pitfalls of either restrictive dieting or rage, I would suggest that as health partners we develop a strategy that incorporates the eating and enjoyment of healthy food along with reasonable mobility. Right now for myself, unfortunately, most movement is painful and a moderate loss of weight over a long time coupled with a slow strengthening of my muscles to carry my weight may be what the doctor and patient ordered.

3. Obesity obscures diagnosis through generalization and shame

Before directly addressing the issue of weight, I would like to evaluate my current health. This is difficult since obesity can mask real health problems. I am not quick to discuss my health due to shame. Lifting layers of fat to examine body orifices is a humiliating procedure for some fat people. I call this the "untouchability" factor. The social shame coupled with the body image issues of obese people are not unlike the leper whose disease keeps people well away.

I have a psychodynamic theory why this might be the case. *Many, but not all,* obese people have developed obesity as a response to abuse or denigration by their family. The necessary medical examination may bring back the body's memory of abuse, real or symbolic. This factor would be doubly relevant if the sexual organs are part of the problem. If patients perceive the demeanor of a physician as uncaring, detached, or in a hurry, this unconsciously cues patients they are being treated inhumanely.

The most obvious thing about my health is my size but weight may not be what brings me to the doctor's office on every occasion. For instance, if my ankle hurts it may be the tremendous weight I carry on my feet, or it might be anything from a small fracture to a sprain. The usual response to an obese person complaining of sore ankles is the stern admonition to lose weight and the pain will go away. However, any foot doctor will have to acknowledge that even thin people can have foot problems.

Another example is genetic heart disease. Although obesity is a contributing factor to heart problems, if several members of the family have died of a heart attack then there is at least one reason beyond obesity for causation. This is true in my case. Three people in my family have had heart problems, yet I have been given the impression by many doctors that any heart pain I sense is the result of obesity alone. If a doctor is distracted by my weight, he is not likely to search for other explanations. Obesity obscures diagnosis.

Often the overall effect of patient shame is concealment of important medical data needed for thorough examinations. For instance, if under one of those layers of fat lies a mole or some other growth, it may go undetected. Hemorrhoids in many people go unreported, but in the obese, due to the physical and psychological discomfort, they are more often unacknowledged.

4. A key to health partnerships involves respectful trusting relationships between non-prejudiced doctors and non-defensive patients.

As much as I would like to enter with you in a partnership toward health, the principles above must be respected, discussed and acknowledged. If you have read this far, I am confident that you have goodwill and are concerned with my well-being. It is central to my view that the relationship that we establish for the betterment of my health is characterized by mutual respect. Patients, obese or otherwise, are no longer passive in their health care. So I look forward in improving my health along with you, and enabling you to deal more effectively with me as your patient. Undoubtedly, my weight will be a contributing factor to many of the ailments I come to you with, but with the above principles in mind, I think we have made a great first step toward partnership.

Respectfully Yours,

Arthur P. Patterson

Arthur P. Patterson holds a masters degree in Spiritual Theology and Literature, and has worked as a pastor, spiritual director, counselor and writer for eighteen years. He is presently facilitator of Watershed. For additional copies or to personally respond: e-mail: taliesin@kwanza.com or write: 694 Victor St, Winnipeg, Man., Canada R3E 1Y5

REFERENCES

1. Cassell JA. Social anthropology and nutrition: A different look at obesity in America. *J Am Diet Assoc.* 1995; 95:424-427.

2. Robison JI, Hoerr SL, Petersmarck KA, Andersen JV. Redefining success in obesity intervention: The new paradigm. *J Am Diet Assoc.* 1995; 95:422-423.

3. Begley CE. Government should strengthen regulation of the weight loss industry. *J Am Diet Assoc.* 1991; 91:1255-1257.

4. America's Weight Problem: What Are We Doing About It? *Calorie Control Commentary.* 1996; 18:1-2.

5. Kuczmarski R, Flegal K, Campbell S, Johnson C. Increasing prevalence of overweight among US adults: the NHANES surveys 1960 to 1991. *JAMA.* 1994; 272: 205-211.

6. National Institutes of Health Technology Assessment Conference. Methods for voluntary weight loss and control. *Ann Intern Med.* 1992; 116:942-949.

7. Berg FM, ed. *The Health Risks of Weight Loss.* Hettinger, ND: Healthy Living Institute; 1995.

8. Brownell KD, Rodin J. The dieting maelstrom: Is it possible and advisable to lose weight? *Am Psychol.* 1994; 49:781-791.

9. Garner DM, Wooley SC. Confronting the failure of behavioral and dietary treatments for obesity. *Clin Psychol Rev.* 1991; 11:729-780.

10. *Top Ten Reasons to Give Up Dieting.* Mt. Marian, NY: International No Diet Coalition, 1996.

11. Yanovski SZ. A practical approach to treatment of the obese patient. *Arch Fam Med.* 1993; 2:309-316.

12. Wadden TB, Van Itallie TB, eds. *Treatment of the Seriously Obese Patient.* New York, NY: Guilford Press. 1992:3-32.

13. Pi-Sunyer FX. Short-term medical benefits and adverse effects of weight loss. *Ann Intern Med.* 1993; 119:722-726.

14. Andres R, Muller MS, Sorkin JD. Long-term effects of change in body weight on all-cause mortality: A review. *Ann Intern Med.* 1993; 119:737-743.

15. Troiano RP, Frongello EA, Sobal J, Levitsky DA. The relationship between body weight and mortality: A quantitative analysis of combined information from existing studies. *Int J Obes.* 1996; 20:63-75.

16. Berg FM. New guidelines given for "healthy weight." *Hthy Wt J.* 1996; 10:53-54, 57.

17. Berg F. Vitality promotes healthy weights, healthy concepts across Canada. *Obes & Hlth.* 1995; 9:50-52.

18. *Living in a Healthy Body: A New Look at Health and Weight.* San Bruno, CA: Krames Communication; 1995.

19. Hirschmann JR, Munter CH. *When Women Stop Hating Their Bodies.* New York, NY: Fawcett Columbine; 1995.

20. Allison DB, ed. *Handbook of Assessment Methods for Eating Behaviors and Weight-Related Problems.* Newbury Park, CA: Sage Publications; 1995.

21. Ciliska D. *Beyond Dieting: Psychoeducational interventions for chronically obese women.* New York, NY: Brunner/Mazel; 1990.

22. Carrier KM, Steinhardt MA, Bowman S. Rethinking traditional weight management programs: A three-year follow-up evaluation of a new approach. *J Psych.* 1994; 128:517-535.

23. Polivy J, Herman C. Undieting: A program to help people stop dieting. *Int J of Eating Disord.* 1992; 11:261-268. 24. Omichinski L, Harrison KR. Reduction of dieting attitudes and practices after participation in a non-diet lifestyle program. *J Can Diet Assoc.* 1995; 56:81-85.

25. Roughan P, Seddon E, Vernon-Roberts J. Long-term effects of a psychologically based group programme for women preoccupied with weight and eating behaviour. *Int J of Obes.* 1990; 14:135-147.

26. Armstrong D, King A. 'Demand feeding' as diabetes treatment. *Obes & Hlth.* 1993; 7:109-110, 115.

27. Steinhardt MA, Nagel L. Effectiveness of the Overcoming Overeating approach to the problem of compulsive eating. In Hirschmann JR, Munter CH. *When Women Stop Hating Their Bodies.* New York, NY: Fawcett Columbine; 1995: 329-345.

28. Corporation professionelle des dietetistes du Quebec. The treatment of obesity: Facilitate without harm. *Obes & Hlth.* 1993; 7:92.

29. *Merriam-Webster's Collegiate Dictionary, Tenth Edition.* Springfield, MA: Merriam-Webster, Inc; 1994.

30. *Reaching Consumers with Meaningful Health Messages: Putting the Dietary Guidelines into Action.* Dietary Guidelines Alliance; 1996.

31. Polivy J. Psychological consequences of food restriction. *J Am Diet Assoc.* 1996; 96:589-594.

32. Berg F. *Children and Teens in Weight Crisis: Guidelines for Healthy Change.* Hettinger, ND: Healthy Weight Journal; 1995.

33. *Mirror, Mirror: A Resource Guide for Helping Adolescents Develop a Positive Body Image and Maintain a Healthy Weight.* Chicago, IL: National Live Stock and Meat Board; 1992.

34. Satter E. *How to Get Your Kid to Eat ... But Not Too Much: From Birth to Adolescence.* Palo Alto, CA: Bull Publishing; 1987.

35. Hirschmann JR, Zaphiropoulos L. *Solving Your Child's Eating Problems: A Completely New Approach to Raising Children Free of Food and Weight Problems.* New York, NY: Fawcett Columbine; 1990.

36. Omichinski L. *Teens and Diets: No Weigh.* Canada: HUGS International, Inc; 1995.

37. Elam P, Kimbrell D. Size, lies and measuring tape. *Cog and Behav Prac.* 1995; 2: 233-248.

38. Goodman WC. *The Invisible Woman: Confronting Weight Prejudice in America.* Carlsbad, CA: Gurze Books; 1995.

39. *Guidelines for health care providers in dealing with fat patients.* Sacramento, CA: NAAFA.

40. Fraser L. Should you treat obesity? *Hippocrates.* 1993; May: 24, 26-27.

Moving Away From Diets A Professional Perspective

Despite overwhelming agreement on the failure of diets to promote lasting change and growing evidence of potentially dangerous physical and psychological consequences, weight-related research and intervention continue to focus on the promotion of weight loss through dietary restriction. And despite almost universal recidivism following weight-loss programs and an epidemic of dangerous eating disorders, people continue to spend billions of dollars yearly on weight loss products and services.

As a male practitioner, who has been helping people with weight-related concerns for more than 10 years, I am deeply troubled by this continued investment in a clearly failed and potentially harmful approach. Our culture's unrelenting obsession with thinness has spawned a pervasive prejudice that causes tremendous suffering and social isolation for individuals of size. This is particularly damaging for young girls and women who are pressured to divert significant proportions of their energy and resources to the pursuit of ideals of body shape and size that are, for the vast majority, neither achievable nor healthy. Indeed, women of all sizes suffer from an intense fear of fat that plays havoc with their self-esteem and promotes disordered eating and exercise behaviors. Men suffer as well by participating in a culture that defines the worth of more than one half of its population in terms of physical appearance, rather than by the recognition of truly meaningful qualities such as honesty, compassion, and love.

This tremendous pressure to be thin is driven by diet, fashion, cosmetics, fitness, and the pharmaceutical industries that reap tremendous financial rewards by promoting unattainable expectations, particularly for women. In addition, many obesity researchers have economic links to this so called "diet-pharmaceutical-industrial complex," creating powerful incentives for maintaining the status quo.

We must look more closely at obesity research. For example, in the recent Nurses study, though the data showed no increase in health risk for women with BMI's between 21 and 27, somehow the message emerged that a BMI of 19 was the ideal for which women should strive. This is a level used by eating disorder experts as an indicator of anorexia nervosa.

Studies indicate that health professionals are often extremely prejudicial in their treatment of larger individuals. The nondiet approach offers practitioners an alternative for compassionate, health-enhancing care. This approach encourages self-acceptance by honoring the natural diversity in body shape and size, and exposing societal prejudice and discrimination against larger individuals. It promotes the benefits of physical activity by encouraging social, pleasure-driven movement. And it helps people to reconnect eating to internally driven hunger, appetite and satiety cues, leading to a more normal, peaceful, relationship with food.

By breaking the endless cycle of weight loss and regain, this approach can help to stop the waste of valuable resources that results from our cultural obsession with thinness. The goal is to help people make positive changes to improve the quality of their lives regardless of weight status. The end result will be a culture that is less judgmental and more truly diverse with more individuals who lead healthy, fulfilled lives by honoring and caring for the bodies they already have.

Jon Robison, PhD, Health Education & Exercise Physiology, MS, Human Nutrition
Executive Co-Director, Michigan Center for Preventive Medicine
Adjunct Assistant Professor, Department of Physical Education & Exercise Science, Michigan State University

2

Loving the Body You Have: Size Acceptance

> *I'm not trying to prove that every big person is a paragon of perfection, civility, beauty, or even good health, but rather that weight prejudice is predicated on the fantasy that the thin person is all of these things, and that therefore any and all harassment and discrimination against the fat person is entirely justified* (1).

WEIGHTY MATTERS: WHAT IS FATISM?

Prejudice against large people, sometimes called fatism, is one of the last, socially permissible forms of bigotry in America today. Fatism manifests in dozens of forms: from name calling in schools and on the streets to overt discrimination in college admissions, job applications, and health care treatment. Size discrimination is oppressive and pervasive, and it has profound, lasting effects on children and adults (1,2). As professionals who seek to enhance the health of large people, we must be sensitive to the devastating effects of fatism, and be willing to examine our own assumptions, beliefs and behaviors. The National Association to Advance Fat Acceptance (NAAFA) checklist (Figure 2-A) developed by Susan Kano (3) is an easy way to assess attitudes. We must begin to make changes that support "the physical and emotional health of fat people through personal and social change (3)."

Myths About Being Fat

Fatism and myths about fat people can cloud our view of their health and food issues. Recognizing the myths and misconceptions is one step to providing high quality health care to people of all sizes. Dr. Barbara Altman Bruno, NAAFA's Mental Health Advisor reminds us that, "Fat people have been reminded constantly that they are faulty and do not fit in (4)." The following fat myths and corresponding realities are adapted from the NAAFA publications (4,5):

Myth #1: All fat people are compulsive eaters.
   Reality: Some fat people (as well as some thin people) are compulsive eaters; some are not. Since compulsive overeating can occur in response to restrictive dieting, people who diet are at risk for bingeing. While most fat people, especially women, have dieted for years or even decades, some have developed compulsive eating problems. Once dieting stops, compulsive behavior often begins to heal and eating patterns normalize.

Myth #2: Fat people become fat from overeating and being lazy. They can become thin by dieting and exercising.

continued on page 19

Figure 2-A

Fat Acceptance Behavior Assessment

1= never 2= rarely 3= occasionally 4= frequently 5= daily

How often do you:

1. make negative comments about your fatness _____
2. make negative comments about someone else's fatness _____
3. directly or indirectly support the assumption that no one should be fat _____
4. say something that presumes being fat is unhealthy _____
5. say something that presumes being thin is healthy _____
6. say or assume that someone is "looking good" because she or he lost weight _____
7. say something that presumes that a fat person wants to lose weight _____
8. say something that presumes that a fat person should lose weight _____
9. say something that presumes that fat people eat too much or "the wrong things" _____
10. disapprove of someone for gaining weight _____
11. assume something is "wrong" when someone gains weight _____
12. admire weight loss dieting or rigidly controlled eating _____
13. admire compulsive or excessive exercising _____
14. tease someone about his or her eating (habits or choices) _____
15. criticize someone's eating to a third person ("so-and-so eats way too much junk") _____
16. discuss food in terms of "good or bad" _____
17. talk about "being good" and "being bad" in reference to eating behavior _____
18. say something that presumes being thin is better (or more attractive) than being fat _____
19. comment that you don't wear a certain style because "it makes you look fat" _____
20. comment that you love certain clothing because it "makes you look thin" _____
21. participate in a "fat joke" by telling one, or laughing, or smiling at one _____
22. support the diet industry by buying their services or products _____
23. undereat or exercise obsessively to maintain an unnaturally low weight _____
24. encourage someone to let go of guilt _____
25. encourage or admire self acceptance and self-appreciation or love _____
26. encourage someone to feel good about his or her body as is _____
27. openly admire a fat person's appearance _____
28. openly admire a fat person's character, personality, or actions _____
29. oppose or challenge fatism verbally _____
30. oppose or challenge fatism in writing _____
31. challenge or voice disapproval of a "fat joke" _____
32. challenge myths about fatness and eating _____
33. compliment ideas, behavior, character, etc. more often than appearance _____
34. support organizations which advance fat acceptance (with your time or money) _____

Behaviors # 1-23 are not helpful or downright harmful to a heavy person's mental health. Look over your 3-4-5 answers to isolate areas that need improvement. Strive to avoid these and similar behaviors in the future.

Behaviors # 24-34 show fat acceptance and are consistent with the size acceptance movement. Reread items where you marked 1 or 2; make a list of realistic goals for increasing supportive behavior.

Adapted from survey by Susan Kano for National Association to Advance Fat Accetance
Used with permission.

Reality: Some people gain weight from eating too much and moving too little. However, some large people gain weight eating no more than thin people. Others maintain high weights eating no more than thin people. If someone has become fat from a combination of overeating and under exercising, *their size may diminish* as they eat less and exercise more. Nevertheless, they may never become thin, unless their genetics program their bodies to be thin.

Myth #3: Fat people are avoiding or covering their sexuality.
Reality: Some people may use fatness to protect themselves sexually. However, this is an individual issue. Many large people are comfortable with their sexuality, are sexually active, and enjoy healthy sexual relationships.

Myth #4: Most fat women have been sexually abused when they were young.
Reality: It is estimated that 25 to 30% of *all* women have been sexually abused. One cannot assume any direct correlation between body size and a history of physical or sexual abuse.

Myth #5: Fat people lack willpower.
Reality: Most fat people in our culture have spent years dieting, and many have lost and regained hundreds or even thousands of pounds. The human body interprets very low calorie diets as starvation, which naturally can result in both physical and psychological urges to overeat or even binge. This serves to protect the body from too drastic a drop in body size or nutritional status. Years of starvation diets may reduce muscle mass thus lowering an individual's metabolic rate so weight loss becomes far more difficult.

Myth #6: Inside every fat person is a thin person trying to get out.
Reality: Given the prejudice which confronts fat people in our society, most large people would like to be thinner. We cannot assume any fat person can become thin with current treatments. Genetics, age, and dieting history all impact body size and shape. With the right treatment, large people can heal eating problems or exercise resistance, and lead fulfilled, happy, and healthy lives.

Myth #7: Fat people are ugly.
Reality: Beauty is a learned concept and the cultural norm of beauty changes over time. At the turn of the century, the leading American sex symbol, Lillian Russell, weighed over 200 pounds. Even Marilyn Monroe, sex symbol of the 1950's, is overweight by today's standards. The media, advertisers, and the diet industry tend to set the standards of beauty in today's Western societies. In other countries worldwide, possessing an ample body ranges from a revered sign of affluence to a neutral issue with little social meaning.

To help combat myths and insure that your practice, programs, and materials are size friendly, review Figure 2-B on page 20, "Guidelines for Health Care Providers in Dealing with Fat Patients."

SIZE ACCEPTANCE
All the pain and oppression and torturous silence my body had had to bear for so many years--the pain of not being trusted, the pain of not being used, the pain of being fed beyond fullness, the pain of being starved--all came screaming out. And we cried--my body, my spirit, my mind--until we became one (6).

Deciding to stop dieting is a step more and more people are willing to take. Baby boomers have been "watching their weight" and dreaming of guilt-free chocolate cake and buns of steel for 10, 20, 30, or

continued on page 21

Figure 2-B

Guidelines for Health Care Providers in Dealing with Fat Patients

PHILOSOPHY OF HEALTH CARE

Attitude

As a responsible health care professional, you should acknowledge each of your patients as an individual. This is especially true for fat patients, who may avoid health care when they feel they are only perceived as being fat, and that the knee-jerk treatment for any problem is "lose weight." If they *could* lose weight, many *would* have done so by now.

While fat people are often not taken seriously by health care providers, please treat them with gentleness, tact and concern.   Remember that many have had years of negative experiences and some have been denied treatment, or given inappropriate treatment because they are fat.

Weighing Patients

- Do not automatically weigh your fat patients, unless there is a compelling reason to do so.
- If weighing is necessary, ensure that it takes place in a private setting, and not in the presence of other patients and staff.
- The fat patient's weight should be recorded silently, free of any commentary.

MEDICAL TREATMENT

Medical Procedures

- Have several sizes of blood pressure cuffs available. Using a small cuff on a fat patient can cause false readings.
- Have longer needles and tourniquets available to draw blood from your fat patients.
- Your lavatory should have a seat that is split in front, to enable fat patients to more easily hold urine specimen cups in place. A urine specimen collection device with a handle is preferable.

Diagnosing Medical Problems

- Do not automatically assume that the cause of your fat patient's condition is his or her weight. (As one patient had to remind her physician, "Don't let my weight get in the way of my credibility.")
- Remember to perform the same diagnostic tests on your fat patients as you would on your patients of average size.

Treating Medical Problems

- Do not insist your fat patient lose weight before receiving treatment for conditions that are not weight related.
- Demonstrate care in ordering medication dosages. Some fat patients react sensitively to small dosages of some drugs, while other drugs require a higher dosage, due to the patient's higher weight.

ACCOMMODATIONS

Waiting Room

- Have several sturdy armless chairs in your waiting room. Chairs with arms often cannot accommodate a fat person.
- There should be six to eight inches of space between chairs.
- Sofas should be firm and high enough to ensure that your fat patients can easily rise. Exceptionally low and soft sofas can be a nightmare for the fat patient.

Examination Room

- Examining tables should be wide, and bolted to the floor or wall, so that the table does not tip forward when your fat patient sits on the end.
- Provide a sturdy stool for fat patients to assist them in getting on the examining table.
- Provide super-large examining gowns for your fat patients.

National Association to Advance Fat Accetance. Adaptation. Used with permission.

even 40 years. Many are sick and tired of the rituals of restrictive dieting, compulsive exercising, and body bashing. *They are ready to just say no to diets.*

The next step is a tough one. It is a struggle for die-hard weight watchers to accept that body perfection is not possible. After buying the "thin is best" myth for decades, it can be a painful grieving process to grapple with the reality of being in a larger than acceptable body. In our culture, even average size men and women struggle with negative body image issues, but large women and children of both genders suffer most from our distorted goals.

Whatever the client's size, no matter how difficult the process, self-acceptance is essential. Feeling good about their bodies and trusting internal signals are essential for several reasons:

1. The close connection between mind and body is increasingly recognized as a critical component of overall health. Only with self-acceptance can your mind and body really connect with each other.

2. It is tough to take good care of something or someone a person hates. When clients are dissatisfied with their bodies, it is hard to take care of them, even in simple ways like wearing a seat belt or brushing their teeth.

3. Self-care is necessary for optimal health and well-being because no one is going to make all the healthy choices for another individual. As adults, clients have to care enough about themselves to want what is best for their health.

4. Making healthy choices is much easier when a person has a sense of peace and wholeness. Making positive choices is difficult, if not impossible, when clients are busy yelling about how "fat," "disgusting," and "out of control" they are.

SOCIETY INFLUENCES OUR OPINIONS

> *Our culture is swept up in a web of peculiar and distorted beliefs about beauty, health,*
> *virtue, eating, and appetite. We have elevated the pursuit of a lean, fat free body to a*
> *new religion. It has a creed: "I eat right, watch my weight, and exercise (7)."*

Numerous books expose and explore the U.S. cultural obsession with thin bodies, especially for women (1,8,9). If we are going to help people learn to accept, trust, and care for their bodies, we must confront the impact of the beauty myth and weight prejudice on clients. Confronting the issues is essential because size acceptance is only possible when we reject the myths and recognize that *no one deserves to be discriminated against because of the shape of their skin.*

Transforming our individual and collective body image is difficult. The media bombard us with "thin is good" and "fat is bad." Anorectic models are the norm on magazine covers, while nearby headlines and articles relentlessly urge us to lose weight and get in shape (10).

Nearly all role models portrayed in the media are thin, young, and beautiful. The diversity of Americans, in terms of color, shape and size, is clearly not reflected in the images that surround us. In fact, the average U.S. woman is 5'4" tall, weighs 142 pounds, and wears a size 12 to 14, while the average fashion model is 5'9" tall, weighs 110 pounds, and wears a size 6-8 (10). The 30 million U.S. women who wear a size 16 or greater are nearly invisible in the mainstream media and the fashion press.

The current cult of hard bodies and fat free foods is so universal that we have to search to find support for alternative views. In addition to the media messages, there are family, friends, colleagues, and health providers who are more than willing to dole out endless tips on how to "shape up." Being assertive against this tide of judgmental and punitive advice is like swimming upstream. One of the best reasons for talking about size acceptance in groups is that people get support for gentler approaches to food and fitness.

NAAFA's Mental Health Advisor, therapist Barbara Altman Bruno summarizes it by suggesting, "you have to disagree to have a great life (11)." For clients to accept themselves, they may have to disagree with society's stereotypes with some health warnings, with their family's shame about fat, and with the discrimination against overweight people. Sometimes bucking the tide is painful, but, according to Dr. Bruno (and many others), if you get a great life, it's worth it!

HOW CAN PEOPLE LEARN TO LOVE THEIR BODIES?

If you want to be fat, healthy and fit, do what healthy and fit people do. Eat healthfully, be physically and mentally active, get appropriate health care, and enjoy yourself. If you want love in your life, find ways to be loving to those already in your life, including yourself (11).

The Basic Tenets of Health at Every Size are outlined in Figure 2-C (12). The most basic principle of all is quite simple: ***Healthy, beautiful bodies come in all sizes, shapes, and weights.*** Accepting this fact is one more way of embracing the strength and power inherent in human diversity.

People can learn to love and trust their bodies. Learning to listen and respond to internal signals works best as a gentle journey, taken one step at a time. It is a process that health providers can facilitate in many ways, always remembering that "This stuff takes time (13)."

In talking about the process of size and self-acceptance in *"Nothing to Lose: A Guide to Sane Living in a Large Body"* (13), Dr. Cheri Erdman suggests that everyone needs support for changing their mind about their body. Support for size acceptance can come from dozens of directions: books, magazines, and videos; educational handouts; clothing catalogs and stores; peer groups and movement classes; counseling and therapy (talk, art and movement); and size friendly professionals.

STAGES OF SIZE ACCEPTANCE PROCESS

The process of size acceptance has several stages. Erdman describes these stages as: pre-acceptance, initial acceptance, midpoint acceptance, and decisive acceptance (13). Bruno likens them to the stages of recovery that are necessary to empower people to take control of their lives and make their way in a world that is not always welcoming (11). The four stages suggested by Bruno are:

1. Recognize the myths about fat and the realities about diets.
2. Claim responsibility for health and begin to listen to internal messages.
3. Redefine personal goals.
4. Get involved.

Whatever labels you choose to use, these stages define the steps you can take to help people learn to love their bodies. There is not just one way to go through the process. Some steps will take longer than others. Fortunately, there are dozens of ways you can facilitate size acceptance in your practice. Here are a few possible strategies you can use to help clients accept themselves and learn to move away from diets.

1. Recognize the myths about fat and the realities about diets.

- **Outline the facts about the frustration and failure of traditional weight loss diets.** Use one of the handouts, or prepare your own sheet with the facts about diet failure rates and the risk of weight loss. Ask clients to share their dieting histories and confirm that their experience is a universal one (they are not personal failures, dieting is a failure based activity).

- **Discuss the shameful and painful things that have been done or said to large people in the name of "health."** Invite your clients to write or talk about their personal experiences with

Figure 2-C

BASIC TENETS OF HEALTH AT EVERY SIZE

- Human beings come in a variety of sizes and shapes. We celebrate this diversity as a positive characteristic of the human race.

- There is no ideal body size, shape, or weight that every individual should strive to achieve.

- Every body is a good body.

- Self-esteem and body image are strongly linked. Helping people feel good about their bodies and about who they are, can help motivate and maintain healthy behaviors.

- Appearance stereotyping (beauty-is-good, homely-is-bad) is inherently unfair to the individual because it is based on superficial factors that the individual has little or no control over.

- We respect the bodies of others even though they might be quite different from our own.

- Each person is responsible for taking care of his or her body.

- Good health is not defined by body size; it is a state of physical, mental, and social well-being.

- People of all sizes and shapes can reduce their risk of poor health by adopting a healthy lifestyle.

Conclusion

Health promotion programs should celebrate the benefits of a healthy lifestyle. Programs should be sensitive to size diversity. They should promote body satisfaction, and the achievement of realistic and attainable health goals without regard to weight change.

Used with permission.

Developed by Dietitians and Nutritionists who are advocates of size acceptance; their efforts coordinated by Joanne P. Ikeda, MA, RD, Nutrition Education Specialist, Department of Nutritional Sciences, University of California, CA 94720-3104. Comments regarding these tenets may be sent to <jikeda@garnet.berkeley.edu>.

in their own family, at school and work, and in daily life. Suggest they read *"The Invisible Woman"* (listed in this chapter), and discuss their reactions and their feelings about discrimination.

- **Share common experiences, beliefs, and myths about food and eating, weight and size, diet, and exercise.** Help your clients identify their personal belief systems about weight, food, and exercise. Discuss how the common myths have developed and begin to debunk their misconceptions. Identify the beliefs and myths that are obstacles or barriers to the healthy lifestyle they want.

- **Read materials that discuss the historic and cultural context of weight and food issues.** Suggest your clients read *"The Beauty Myth"* or one of many books listed in the resource section of this chapter. Share (through books, postcards or museum visits) artwork with changing images of beauty through the centuries. Compare how body type is viewed today versus in other times and countries.

- **Get rid of the scale and choose to weigh only when medically necessary.** Discuss clients' relationship with the scale--when, how often, and why they weigh themselves. Help them wean away from the power of scale. Discuss the situations when weight measurements may be medically necessary (e.g. anesthesia, pregnancy, cardiac failure). Role play situations where someone asks clients their weight or to step on the scale to be weighed (i.e. physician's office, driver's license bureau, etc.).

2. Claim responsibility for health and begin to listen to internal messages.

- **Develop new messages to replace negative ones from family, friends, colleagues, professionals, and media.** Have clients make a list of negative comments regarding their size, weight, or shape, including ones like "my mother always said _____" and "my coworkers always talk about _____." Make contrasting lists of new, positive, empowering messages like "I love my legs because they help carry me through every day."

- **Choose to ignore or confront the name calling and negative labels from people and begin to "trust your guts."**

- **Role play situations that involve insulting and discriminating messages from strangers.** Discuss the negative and hostile feelings that are natural reactions. Brainstorm positive new ways to handle the situations and feelings.

- **Watch the process of size acceptance and begin to discuss the changes with people you know.**

- **Encourage clients to create a journal or artwork about the process of acceptance.** Suggest they write or draw about the thoughts, feelings, difficulties, and changes as they experience them (see *"SomeBody to Love"* listed at the end of this chapter). Plan ways they can share these changes with significant people in their lives (parents, siblings, partners, children, friends, and colleagues as appropriate).

- **Read magazines that feature beautiful, healthy people of all sizes, wearing all kinds of clothes, and doing all sorts of interesting things.**

- **Use magazines, newspapers, and newsletters to identify the usual messages about size, weight, and shape in the mainstream press.** Encourage clients to get rid of materials that make size acceptance more difficult. Introduce alternative media like *Radiance* and *BBW* (listed in the references at the end of this chapter) and discuss which mainstream magazines have the most accurate information and advice about nutrition and physical activity.

- **Explore new options in work and play to see which jobs, classes, and activities provide the most pleasure and satisfaction.** Discuss all the aspects of total health--physical, mental, emotional, and spiritual. Encourage the exploration of completely new and different activities or return to those that were important in childhood ("I used to love to paint as a child but I have not done anything artistic in years.") Provide assistance in overcoming barriers to new activities, like special aerobics classes or swim schedules for large people.

3. Redefine personal goals.

- **Create new definitions and affirmations of self.** Assist clients in transforming body image by changing the words they use to describe themselves. Use activities like talking to a mirror or positive self talk to a mirror image (see *Transforming Body Image* listed at the end of this chapter) to move from negative judgmental messages through neutral descriptors to empowering affirmations (from "fat slob" to "round woman" to "gorgeous Ruebenesque figure" or "fit and active"). Help them feel comfortable with concepts like, "I am fat and fulfilled,"or "I am large and happy and healthy," or in some cases, "I am normal in size."

- **Learn to assert individual needs for comfort and safety.** Discuss situations where clients may feel intimidated because of their size or weight, like airplane seating, clothing stores or fitness centers. Role play ways to be assertive in the face of overt or covert discrimination ("may I have a seatbelt extender, please"). Identify ways their lives could be more comfortable and active with adapted equipment (wide, padded bicycle seats) or clothing (walking shoes with extra insoles).

- **Choose friends, doctors, and therapists who practice size acceptance and support health without focusing on weight loss.** Assist clients in identifying whether their health care providers and friends are size friendly and supportive of their self-acceptance. Provide handouts or other materials that can be used to educate the significant people in their lives. Discuss situations where it may be appropriate to seek other providers or move to other friendships.

- **Shop size friendly stores and catalogs to choose beautiful, comfortable, fashionable clothes that fit individual lifestyles.** Help clients get rid of clothes that do not fit or are painful reminders of failed diets. Discuss possible donations, trading, or sale of clothing to minimize financial impact. Identify resources (books, magazines, stores, or consultants) to develop a personal fashion style based on both appearance and comfort for a variety of activities.

- **Invest time, energy and money in self-care rather than the diet industry, indulge with haircuts, manicures, massage, and complete rest and relaxation.** Brainstorm a variety of stress reduction and self-care activities appropriate for your clients' time and financial resources. Identify those activities that provide the biggest "bang" for their self-care "buck." Help clients give themselves permission for self-care and relaxation, even when they think they are undeserving.

4. Get involved.

- **Join groups and organizations that promote size esteem and support diversity.** Provide clients with lists of local groups and national organizations (like NAAFA) that promote size acceptance. Establish a support, education, or treatment group for clients and other community members.

- **Participate in events to make a statement about size acceptance.** Encourage your clients to organize or participate in size acceptance events, like International No-Diet Day (May 6th). Assist local planners in designing events to educate people about issues related to fatism, the dangers of dieting, and eating disorder prevention.

- **Share success stories.** Empower clients to share their stories with others who struggle with similar issues. Encourage them to write letters, articles, or books, talk to churches, colleagues, or community groups, or go on TV or radio. Help them have fun with fashion shows or fitness events that feature people of all sizes, who look and feel great.

- **Support positive portrayals of beautiful bodies in all shapes, sizes, and colors.** Suggest clients monitor the media for products, people, and institutions that promote size acceptance and a nondiet approach to health and fitness. Encourage them to write letters or make calls to both compliment positive images and complain about negative ones.

- **Speak out against weight prejudice, harassment, and discrimination.** Inspire clients to promote size acceptance and to denounce fatism wherever it exists. Help them overcome the natural fear of speaking against a societal norm. Connect them with people and resources to support their involvement in whatever form they feel comfortable.

TOOLS and RESOURCES

I believe that all women are goddesses, and goddesses come in all shapes and sizes. My clothing is designed to help real women find both the goddess within them and celebrate their own style (15).

Ten years ago the resources available to promote size acceptance were rare. Now there are dozens of books and videos, some of which are beginning to challenge the diet best sellers. This section includes an extensive list of resources and a camera-ready handout, Loving Your Body, Figure 2-D. The listing in Chapter 1 (*Top Ten Reasons To Give Up Dieting*) also works well for discussing size acceptance, especially for groups.

The following materials will be invaluable as you seek to help clients learn to move away from diets. They are all useful resources for a professional library, but some may be more appropriate than others for your style, situation, and audience. They are divided into two types, professional and general, based on their intended audience. Naturally these divisions are somewhat arbitrary.

Professionals have much to gain by an intimate familiarity with the general resources: increased knowledge, enhanced insight, and new views on familiar topics. Clients, especially those who work in education, health, and technical areas themselves, may want additional data and background information available in the professional resources.

Complete identifying and ordering information accompany each item (listed alphabetically). The prices listed were current as of fall 1996. The brief descriptions are intended to highlight the strengths rather than to provide a comprehensive or critical review of the contents.

Some of these products, and many others, are available in the *Eating Disorders Bookshelf Catalog* from Gurze Books, Box 2238, Carlsbad, CA, 92018. Phone: (800) 756-7533; Fax: (619) 434-5476; Internet: gurze@aol.com. The catalog offers books, video, and audio tapes; subscriptions to *Eating Disorders Review;* a listing of the national organizations; and advertisements for eating disorder programs around the U.S. Free copies of the catalog are available for distribution to clients and colleagues.

Figure 2-D   # LOVING YOUR BODY

Loving your body is hard in our fat phobic, diet obsessed world, but it is worth every ounce of effort you put into it. It means accepting the diversity of human bodies and recognizing no one should be discriminated against because of the shape of their skin. Loving your body means celebrating your uniqueness, your many abilities, and finally making friends with the mirror on your wall.

- Throw away the scale. Weigh yourself only when medically necessary. Even then you can choose to ignore the number if you want.

- Reject fatism in yourself and in others. Recognize that healthy, beautiful bodies come in all shapes and sizes.

- Invest time and money in yourself rather than the diet industry. Spend your money on beautiful clothes, jewelry, haircuts, manicures and massages--not on diets.

- Surround yourself with size friendly people. Choose friends, doctors and therapists who accept the way you are and support the lifestyle changes *you* want to make.

- Stand tall and proud. Straighten your stance, feel energy, strength, and confidence flow from your head to your toes.

- Put your mind in touch with your body. To heighten your confidence and body awareness, look into walking, meditation, t'ai chi, yoga, or movement therapy.

- Clothe your body in beautiful, comfortable clothes that fit *now*. Search out stores and catalogs that cater to people of your size, shape, and fashion sense.

- Join groups that promote size esteem. Look for local and national organizations that provide resources and support the natural diversity of sizes and shapes.

- Read magazines, like *Radiance* and *BBW: Big Beautiful Woman*, that feature large, fashionable women, wearing all types of styles, and doing a variety of activities.

- Be patient with yourself. Old habits die hard. Changes may take awhile to become permanent fixtures in your life.

Developed by Dayle Hayes, MS, RD, Copyright 1996
May be reproduced for educational purposes.

PROFESSIONAL:

Food & Body Connections: Working with Groups to Explore Eating Issues, Body Image, Size Acceptance and Self-care, Sandy Stewart Christian, editor, 1996 (188 p.), Whole Person Associates, 210 West Michigan, Duluth, MN, 55802 (800) 247-6789. ($24.95)

An essential tool for working with groups, this innovative collection includes 36 group processes gathered from U.S. experts. It tackles complex and painful issues (self-esteem, dieting, weight, healthy eating, body image and fitness) with specific exercises that you can reproduce and use in your groups.

Healthy Weight Journal: Research, News and Commentary across the Weight Spectrum, Francie Berg, editor, 402 S. 14th St., Hettinger, ND, 58639 (701) 567-2646. ($59/year for six issues)

Published since 1986, this highly readable journal is dedicated to being a "voice of integrity in a field that has lacked adequate standards." It provides a critical link between research and practical applications and includes a regular column on size acceptance written by experts in the field.

HUGS for Better Health: You Count, Calories Don't, Linda Omichinski, BSc, RD, Box 102A, RR #3, Portage la Prairie, Manitoba, Canada, R1N3A3 (800) 565-4847.

The HUGS program offers a complete line of nondiet products including a workbook, practical cookbook, fitness video, affirmation audio tapes, facilitator kit, and support newsletter. Begun in Canada, the HUGS network now includes five countries. Call for a complete catalog and pricing.

Life's Odyssey ™, Karen Carrier, MEd, Human Solutions, Houston, TX (713) 464-6152.

This is the first holistic health risk appraisal that also promotes the nondiet approach. Other resources to be released soon.

GENERAL RESOURCES:

Amplestuff: Make Your World Fit You (catalog) & *The Ample Shopper* (newsletter), Bill Fabrey, PO Box 116, Bearsville, NY, 12409 (914) 679-3316. (Free catalog and $12/year for four newsletters.)

If someone you know needs an airline seatbelt extender, a large size blood pressure cuff, or a really ample bath towel, look no more. This catalog and newsletter, produced by an ample couple, offer products which improve the quality of life for plus and super size people.

BBW: Big Beautiful Woman--Plus-Size Fashion, Resources and Lifestyles, Janey Milstead, editor, 8484 Wilshire Blvd., Suite 900, Beverly Hills, CA (800) 707-5592. ($9.95/year for four issues.)

This plus size version of a glossy fashion magazine has plenty of color photographs, its own full-size model search, and interviews with large stars of the stage and screen (like Carnie Wilson, Aretha Franklin, Delta Burke, and Roseanne), also included are articles about food, fitness and relationships.

Big Fat Lies: The Truth About Your Weight and Your Health, Glenn Gaesser, PhD, 1996, Fawcett Columbine, NY. ($23.00)

A must read. Exposes the myth that being fat is a life-threatening condition. One of the most complete reviews of the literature published. Witty and informative.

Body Trust: Undieting Your Way to Health and Happiness, Dayle Hayes, MS, RD, 1994 (1-hr video and 30 min. instructor's video), 2110 Overland Ave., Suite. 120, Billings, MT, 59102 (800) 321-9499.

An award winning video, it features a registered dietitian presenting the nondiet approach, along with powerful first person interviews with women who have gotten off the diet roller coaster. It can be used as a kickoff for group discussion or for individual viewing.

Losing It: False Hopes and Fat Profits in the Diet Industry, Laura Fraser, 1988. Plume Books, NY

In this facinating expose, the first book to blow the whistle on the multibillion-dollar diet industry, Fraser shows how doctors, weight loss clinics, and unscrupulous medical researchers all conspire to give false hopes to millions of Americans in exchange for huge profits. ($13.95)

Nothing to Lose: A Guide to Sane Living in a Larger Body, Cheri K. Erdman, PhD, 1995 (189p.), Harper Collins Publishers, New York, NY (800) 331-3761. ($18.00)

Written by a professor/psychotherapist with personal experience in losing and gaining hundreds of pounds, this guide has excellent sections on being and choosing a therapist. The suggestions on the "spiral of acceptance" will be appreciated by women struggling to embrace themselves and their bodies.

One Size Fits All and Other Fables, Liz Curtis Higgs, 1993 (183 p.), Thomas Nelson Publishers, Nashville, TN (800) 762-6565. (also available on audio tape) ($12.99)

Sometimes laughter really is the best medicine, and this book serves up an "appetizing combination of scrumptious honesty and delicious humor." Using surveys, interviews and heartfelt discussions with over 200 plus-size women, the author encourages women to explore the fables which rule their lives.

Radiance: The Magazine for Large Women, Alice Ansfield, editor, PO Box 30246, Oakland, CA, 94604 (510) 482-0680. ($20/year for four issues)

In-depth, insightful articles; beautiful, bountiful fashions; and enlightening, entertaining profiles of large people, this magazine is essential for the thoughtful large woman. Radiance Tours also offers escorted tours for large women to exotic destinations like Alaska, Europe, and the Caribbean.

Self-Esteem Comes In all Sizes: How to Be Happy and Healthy at Your Natural Weight, Carol Johnson, 1995 (331 p.), Gurze Books, Box 2238, Carlsbad, CA 92018. ($18.95)

An entertaining, challenging, respectful self-help guide for size acceptance, this upbeat book enthusiastically emphasizes that size 8 is not a measure of self worth and that "healthy and thin" are not necessarily synonymous. Johnson is committed to the concept that you can look good and feel good at any size.

Size Acceptance & Self-Acceptance: The NAAFA Workbook: A Complete Study Guide, (2nd edition) Sally Smith, editor, 1995, NAAFA, Box 188620, Sacramento, CA 95818.

This comprehensive workbook features professional advice and personal stories on virtually every issue related to self acceptance for fat people. It covers everything from king-size fashion and getting shoes that fit to discrimination in the workplace and finding appropriate health care.

Style is Not a Size: Looking and Feeling Great in the Body You Have, Hara Estroff Marano, 1991 (338 p.), Bantam Books, New York, NY.

Forget the age-old advice on how to "hide your figure flaws" and learn how to look and feel great at any size. With dozens of drawings and lists of clothing sources, this truly informative fashion guide by a former editor of *Vogue* magazine covers everything from underwear to overcoats, from haircuts to shoes. ($15.00)

SomeBody to Love: A Guide to Loving the Body Have, Leslea Newman, 1991 (200 p.), Third Side Press, 2250 W. Farragut, Chicago, IL (312) 271-3029.

The words and writing activities of this encouraging book are designed to help women of all sizes learn to love themselves. The author includes the story of her own eating "dis-ease"; writing exercises for individual and group work; and an anthology of sensitive pieces written by the women in her workshops. ($10.95)

The Invisible Woman: Confronting Weight Prejudice in America, W. Charisse Goodman, 1995 (240 p.), Gurze Books, Carlsbad, CA (800) 756-7533.

This devastating, no-holds barred critique of America's prejudice against fat is a disturbing book, but it is a must-read for medical personnel and mental health providers. With a definite political and feminist perspective, it explores and exposes all aspects of size or weight discrimination and harassment. ($14.95)

Transforming Body Image: Learning to Love the Body You Have, Marcia Germaine Hutchinson, 1985 (149 p.), The Crossing Press, Freedom, CA. (also on audio tape)

This book and tape are packed with worksheets and exercises designed to improve body image and enhance self acceptance. With a feminist viewpoint, they use guided imagery, deeply personal questions, and mirror exercises to reinforce the size acceptance message in dozens of concrete ways. (Book $12.95 and tape $10.95)

When Women Stop Hating Their Bodies, Jane Hirschmann and Carol Munter, 1995 (363 p.), Fawcett Columbine, New York, NY.

In this book, the authors of *Overcoming Overeating* use the voices of hundreds of women to show how "bad body thoughts" are clues to our emotional lives and to describe how women can create an internal caretaker who provides exactly what they need: unconditional acceptance, attention, and empowerment. ($22.50)

ORGANIZATIONS:

Association for the Health Enrichment of Large People (AHELP), P.O. Drawer C, Radford, VA, 24143 (703) 633-1767; Joe McVoy, PhD, Director.

AHELP provides information and support for health professionals who use the nondiet approach in their practices. It offers a quarterly newsletter *(AHELP Forum)* and holds conferences at various locations throughout the United States.

Council on Size and Weight Discrimination. Inc., P.O. Box 305, Mt. Marion, NY, 12456 (914)679-1209; Miriam Berg, President.

The Council is an anti-discrimination activist group which influences public opinion and policy through education, information, networking. It partially funds the *International No Diet Coalition* (same address and phone number), which publishes an extensive directory of nondiet resources.

Largesse: The Network for Size Esteem, P.O. Box 9404, New Haven, CT, 06534-0404 (203) 787-1624; Karen W. Stimson and Richard K. Stimson, Co-Directors.

This is a clearinghouse for resources and information on size diversity empowerment which includes a database, archives and supporting material. They also publish a newsletter *(Size Esteem),* a bimonthly bulletin *(Food for Thought),* and a *Size Diversity Empowerment Kit* ($13.00 includes shipping).

National Association to Advance Fat Acceptance. Inc. (NAAFA), P.O. Box 188620, Sacramento, CA, 95818 (916) 558-6880; Sally E. Smith, Executive Director.

NAAFA is a national organization, with over 50 local US chapters, that works to end discrimination and empower fat people through education, advocacy, and member support, as well as its newsletter.

P.L.E.A.S.E. (Promoting Legislation and Education About Self-Esteem), 91 South Main Street, West Hartford, CT 06107, (203) 521-2515; Lisa Berzins, PhD.

The mission of P.L.E.A.S.E. is to encourage citizens to celebrate diversity and to promote images that foster self-esteem. They publish a newsletter and work on legislative issues, especially in the Northeast U.S.

ELECTRONIC RESOURCES:

UseNet Groups
- **soc.support.fat-acceptance**
- **alt.support.big-folks**

Listservs
- Fat-Acceptance List: To subscribe, send an e-mail message to: **majordomo@world.std.com** and in the body of the message, type: **subscribe fat-acceptance**

- Overcoming Overeating List: To subscribe, send an e-mail message to: **oo-group@eros. columbia. edu** and in the body of the message, type **subscribe <your e-mail address>**

Web Sites
- **Fat!So?:http://cool.infi.net/**
- Largesse : **http://www.fatgir1/com/largesse** or **http://www.fatgirl.factory.net/largesse/**
- NAAFA: **http://naafa.org/**
- Sizism: **http://worcester.Im.com/Imann/feminist/sizism.html/**

For more information on electronic resources, contact Largesse (address and phone above) to order a copy of *Big Bytes--Internet Resources for Fat Folks.*

REFERENCES:

1. Goodman WC. *The Invisible Woman: Confronting Weight Prejudice in America.* Carlsbad, CA: Gurze Books; 1995.
2. Johnson C. Size acceptance: Raising largely positive kids. *Obes and Hlth.* 1993; 7:114, 117.
3. Kano S. *Behavior Assessment: Supporting the physical and emotional health of fat people through personal and social change.* Sacramento, CA: NAAFA.
4. Bruno BA. *Guidelines for therapists who treat fat clients.* Sacramento, CA: NAAFA.
5. Smith S, edition *Size Acceptance & Self-acceptance: The NAAFA Workbook: A Complete Study Guide,* (2nd edition). Sacramento, CA: NAAFA; 1995.
6. Schneider K. Size acceptance: A change of heart brings freedom. *Hlthy Wt J.* 1994; 8:113-114.
7. Seid RP. Too "close to the bone": The historical context for women's obsession with slenderness. In Fallon P, Katzman MA, Wooley SC. *Feminist Perspectives on Eating Disorders.* New York, NY: Guilford Press; 1994:3-16.
8. Wolf N. *The Beauty Myth: How Images of Beauty Are Used Against Women.* New York, NY: William Morrow;   1991.
9. Fallon P, Katzman MA, Wooley SC. *Feminist Perspectives on Eating Disorders.* New York, NY: Guilford Press; 1994.
10. Schneider KS. Mission impossible. *People Magazine.* June 3, 1996; 64-74.
11. Bruno BA. Size acceptance: Disagree and have a great life. *Hlthy Wt J.* 1996; 10: 35-36, 39.
12. Ikeda J. *Basic tenets of health at every size: A size acceptance approach to health promotion.* Berkeley, CA: University of California Cooperative Extension; 1995.
13. Erdman CK. *Nothing to Lose: A Guide to Sane Living in a Larger Body.* New York, NY: Harper Collins; 1995.
14. Dillon L. Designing woman: An interview with Delta Burke. *BBW: Big Beautiful Woman.* 1995; Winter: 21.

Moving Away From Diets
A Professional Perspective

What professional experiences led you to move towards a nondiet paradigm?
The first 12 years of my career in health promotion were spent in a large oil company helping with the startup and ongoing delivery of a multi-million dollar health and fitness program and facility. A funny thing happened along the way however. Several years into our program, our staff began to notice the traditional weight management and exercise programs were NOT helping many people...and in fact, they actually seemed to be hurting some employees. For example, the same people signed up for weight management over and over, and their pattern was always the same. They either dropped out of the program early, or among those who stayed and lost weight, they almost always regained their weight. Each time these folks signed up anew, they were larger. Increasingly, they felt like failures. Of course, it had not occurred to them or us that THEY WERE NOT FAILING...OUR PROGRAMS WERE FAILING THEM!

Even more questionable were the weight loss contests we offered. When we tracked the data for the participants, we found that the employees who participated the most were the ones who gained the most weight over time! These month long competitions mostly encouraged yo-yo dieting. People would starve themselves to quickly lose weight and win a prize. Then they would go back to their habits and needs from before. Nothing had changed.

Last but not least was our cafeteria program, which was full of good intentions. However, we labeled the food with so much nutrition information that people who used to enjoy eating started obsessing about food. Food became "good" or "bad." Some employees appointed themselves "health police" and starting informal judging and shaming of their peers' food choices.

Actually, there is a happy ending to this story! In 1988 we learned about the nondiet approach to resolving eating problems and body dissatisfaction. Our entire staff went through extensive training in this new work. We brought this alternative perspective into every aspect of our health promotion program. We eliminated weight loss programs, weight loss competitions, and stopped labeling all our food. We eliminated weigh-ins and body fat testing as well.

We began teaching people how to stop dieting and instead eat by tuning into their hunger, fullness and body cravings. We promoted size acceptance and started teaching people to stop obsessing about losing weight. People learned to appreciate the bodies they were born with. Most important we began teaching people how to change their lives and stop translating difficulties in life into struggles about food, eating, and weight.

As a health care professional, I no longer present myself as a "role model." Rather than being an "authority" or "expert," I become an ally. I openly let people know I enjoy food...all kinds of food. I also let them know I no longer hold myself to the cultural ideals for beauty. I feel I am literally saving lives as I work. So many people define themselves by their size and appearance, when they learn of size acceptance and the nondiet approach, a whole new person emerges from under so much pain and shame. The new person is confident, independent, happy and no longer feels life has to wait until he or she loses weight.

I know there is tremendous resistance to this new work among both professionals and the public. I think most of the resistance to the nondiet approach is simply a byproduct of the overwhelmingly powerful and unhealthy culture we live in. A culture that only portrays thin people as successful and happy. It is our job to be part of creating a culture of more diverse images. One that creates the freedom people need to choose a lifestyle that embraces enjoyment of food...and respect and appreciation for people of all body sizes.

Karen Carrier, MEd, Co-Director of the Houston Center for Overcoming Overeating, LLC and Co-Founder of Human Solutions, LLC, call (713) 464-6152 for more information.

3
Understanding Disconnected Eating

> *We need to eat to live. This fact makes food a very powerful force and symbol in life. Along with care, warmth, containment, and appropriate stimulation, food is a central aspect of the holding environment that facilitates a baby's growth and development. Hunger, being fed, and satiation are everyone's earliest and most basic experiences of desires, needs, soothing, satisfaction and occur within the first intimate relationships* (1).

Disconnected eating is initiating eating when one is not hungry, restricting food when he or she is hungry (such as in dieting), or continuing to eat past the point of satisfaction or fullness. This could be caused by eating according to a pattern, habit, or time of day, unrelated to hunger. More often, disconnected eating is prompted and perpetuated by emotions like boredom, anxiety, fear, excitement and rejection.

This chapter illustrates the process by which individuals become disconnected from internal hungers, in other words, hunger for physical, emotional, spiritual, social, and mental nourishment. Chapters four, five, and six detail the three facets of HungerWork that heal this disconnection. By integrating these three facets and using the treatment strategies provided, your clients will come to understand and appreciate the origin and function of their problematic eating styles. In turn, they will be free to recreate their own satisfying relationships with food.

DEVELOPMENT OF DISCONNECTED EATING STYLES

> *Starvation and self-imposed dieting appear to result in eating binges once food is available and in psychological manifestations such as preoccupation with food and eating, increased emotional responsiveness and dysphoria, and distractibility. Caution is thus advisable in counseling clients to restrict their eating and diet to lose weight, as the negative sequelae may outweigh the benefits of restraining one's eating* (2).

In a demand-feeding environment, healthy babies naturally self-regulate food intake by eating when hungry and stopping when full, resulting in adequate nutrition to support their growth and health (3,4,5). Many individuals, however, learn or become influenced to disconnect from this ability to self-regulate food intake. Following are three examples of common circumstances that promote disconnection:

1. External Messages
External messages influence or dominate decision-making around food, drowning out the innate cues of hunger and fullness, appetite and satiety (6).

"It is time to eat."

"You must finish the food on your plate before you get dessert."

"How about an ice cream cone to make you feel better?"
"Don't you think you've had enough?"
"If you keep eating like that, you'll get fat."
"I heard it's bad to eat after 7:00 p.m."
"The best thing about fat free food is I can eat as much as I want."
"At least if I eat no fat, I'm safe."

2. Food Deprivation

An individual may diet to lose weight. Health professionals may suggest restricting certain individual foods or amounts of food to manage a nutrition-sensitive disease (i.e. diabetes, renal failure, hyperlipidemia). However, as mentioned earlier, research on the psychological and physical impacts of voluntary and involuntary food restriction shows that people have increased tendencies to focus on food, eat in response to uncomfortable feeling states, and binge eat. These side effects, and others previously mentioned, make it difficult and frightening for individuals to rely on their own judgment and trust the body's cues to prompt a healthful eating style. Most do not recognize when their reliance on internal cues to self-regulate eating dramatically lessens and their relationship with food becomes more problematic.

3. Emotional Eating

Some individuals respond to emotions by eating. Food and the eating process serve to comfort, distract, or "distance" oneself from emotions, as well as express these emotions through food choices and behaviors. Eating in response to emotions interferes with the body's natural physical cues of hunger, fullness, appetite, and satiety. (This emotionally charged relationship with food is discussed in more depth in "The Dieting Cycle" on the following page.)

Regardless which of the above processes the client has experienced, the result is disconnection from internal cues. Additionally, this compromises his or her ability to focus on food as a source of nourishment and satisfaction.

Furthermore, consistently eating beyond the body's fullness and satiety cues may lead to weight gain. If weight gain results, family members, friends, health care providers, teachers, as well as the individual, often become concerned. Our society's culturally and medically accepted norms for body size and weight reinforces this concern. Individuals feel pressured to lose weight. They seek a diet with weight loss as the primary goal.

I still haven't entirely made up my mind that dieting doesn't work, because it does, in the short term. And in the short term it provides real relief while it's working, while I'm feeling like I'm losing weight and looking better and feeling lighter and less lethargic. But, when the inability to stay on the diet comes, as it always does, the feelings of hopelessness and failure are almost overwhelming and unbearable. I guess that's what I remember now about my experiences. I don't want to have to go through that excruciating business again. The closest I've ever come to feeling "peri-suicidal" (not exactly like I would take my own life, but the feeling that this will all be better when I'm dead and don't have to go through this junk again) has been when I've started bingeing my way out of whatever diet I've been trying to adhere to. Lisa G. At-home mom of two little kids. Glendale, CA.

THE APPEAL OF DIETS...THE FEAR OF HUNGER...THE ILLUSION OF CONTROL

Dieting requires the client to disconnect from internal cues. Dieting is an external process. At it's extreme, it is totally removed from any personal connection and unrelated to sensations of hunger and satiety. Dieters learn the only way to stay with the diet is to ignore their hunger. It is not uncommon to see diets promising, "Lose weight without ever feeling hungry." Messages such as these reinforce restrained eaters' fears of hunger. *The restrained eater sees hunger as the barrier to maintaining the diet; giving in to their hunger being a sign of weakness or indulgence.* Dieters commonly believe that "blowing their diet" is due to lack of self-control; a character flaw. They are driven to eat just because of this self-criticism (2).

Staying on a diet while overriding hunger signals and losing weight can give the illusion of control. In actuality, following a regimen that involves restriction or deprivation, can lead to (2,7,8,9):

- preoccupation with food,
- hunger intolerance,
- overeating or binge eating,
- eating in response to emotions,
- weight gain...the absolute opposite results the individual wanted.

So ingrained is dieting that even when it is understood that dieting is not the solution, clients may not know where to turn for help. And clients who wish to return to self-regulated eating may find they are fearful, unable or unsure how to reconnect, interpret, and respond to their bodies' cues.

THE PAINFUL CYCLE OF DEPRIVATION AND COMPENSATORY EATING

The cycle of deprivation and resultant overeating plants seeds of confusion and distrust of internal cues (i.e. hunger and fullness). As a result of restriction, they experience hunger and appetite as overpowering and out of control. They believe succumbing to hunger (eating foods off the plan or off the schedule) is a sign of poor self-control. In actuality, breaking the diet, "cheating" or binge eating is in response to deprivation. This eating behavior is an attempt to reconnect with and respond to the body and return to normal eating.

DEPRIVATION COMBINED WITH EMOTIONAL TRIGGERS TO EAT

Individuals may eat to comfort, distract, and calm themselves. Food deprivation coupled with intense negative emotions can cause overwhelming physical and psychological drives to eat resulting in disconnected eating. This deprivation-driven, emotional eating leaves individuals confused and distressed. They question their motives, desires, and self-discipline because they want foods they either cannot control or are "fattening." They may eat quantities that cause them to be overfull and possibly gain weight. Viewing the "problem" from the clients' perspective explains why they believe stronger resolve is necessary to control this drive to eat.

These people have lost trust in their ability to help themselves and in their bodies' cues. They search for some force outside themselves that will control the drive to eat. They also hope this same solution alleviates the painful emotions that come from feeling chaotic, hopeless, alone, and deprived.

Repeated failures at dieting add to the distress of facing life without having lost weight, and in fact possibly gaining weight. Perhaps the most painful thought for the restrained eater is that the good things in life (love, acceptance, success) may not materialize if they cannot lose weight.

Eventually, they choose a stricter diet to gain control. Negative self-talk emerges because they feel they are to blame for past dieting failures and current "weaknesses." Restriction combined with negative self-talk increases painful emotions they in turn attempt to soothe by eating. This eating can become frenetic, secretive, and vast in quantity. The distress and pain heighten internally. They desire someone or something outside themselves to tell them what to do. The cycle is perpetuated.

THE DIETING CYCLE

The illustration of the dieting cycle (Figures 3-A on page 37 and 3-B on page 39) was developed by Francie White, MA, RD, dietitian, author, and workshop leader in private practice in Santa Barbara, CA (10). We add our explanations to help you understand the process. This Dieting Cycle illustrates the process by which dieting gains momentum, the problems inherent in dieting, and why an alternative is needed. The cycle is described so you can go through it step by step with a client, coordinating the numbers with the illustration.

   Note: Although the cycle is describing a girl, increasingly, boys and men are revealing similar dynamics in relationship to their eating styles, physical activity, body image, size acceptance, and dieting patterns (11).

1. The stick figure represents Alice, a 10-year old girl. (Essentially, she could be a woman graduating from college, a mother in her thirties, a busy male professional, and so on.) She happens to be the kind of person who finds food and the eating experience calming. When she eats, especially carbohydrates, a feeling of relief, an "ahhh" feeling, floods her. Some people tend to find food or the eating experience more calming than others (12). This serves to calm her distressing feelings.

2. Distressing feelings come from deep painful experiences, usually early in childhood or adolescence, but not exclusively from those times. Examples are: experiencing dysfunctional family dynamics, single traumatic incidents (rape, death of a parent, or trauma witness), or ongoing abuse and neglect.

3. Daily life events prompt feelings. Alice starts noticing distress at home, possibly unresolved conflict (overt or covert). Perhaps feelings are not validated. There may be physical or sexual abuse. Feelings she has learned are "unacceptable" and remain unexpressed.

4. She finds when she eats, she feels relief from the distress (all is subconscious at this point).

5. Unfortunately, after the relief from eating dissipates, she finds her stress is still present.

6. To defend herself from the unpleasantness, she must eat again. Initially, this is not a lot of food, but the amount increases as eating becomes her primary coping mechanism.

7. She begins to eat outside hunger and fullness cues (disconnected eating) and consequently begins to gain weight.

8. People who gained weight in other ways enter the cycle here. For example, an individual who: has been sedentary most of his or her life; is genetically heavier than the "norm;" or has been doing some "entertainment eating" (using food to distract). Individuals who consider themselves overweight (and believe they need to lose weight) enter the cycle here, as well.

Note to the health care provider: At this point in the Dieting Cycle, explore the following questions with your client:
   • What is their view of fat? Society's?
   • Is fat unhealthy?
   • How might your life be different if your fat is accepted?

9. This "extra" weight does not need to be a moral issue, except that our culture believes that "fat is bad, fat is unattractive." Viewing fat as bad has significant side effects; weight loss is not one of them. Viewing fat as bad:
   • perpetuates the stereotyping and prejudice of large people,
   • encourages us to value women (and men to a lesser degree) for physical attractiveness, rather than personal qualities,
   • increases food and weight preoccupation and causes associated emotional pain,
   • contributes to the incidence of eating disorders.

Figure 3-A THE DIETING CYCLE

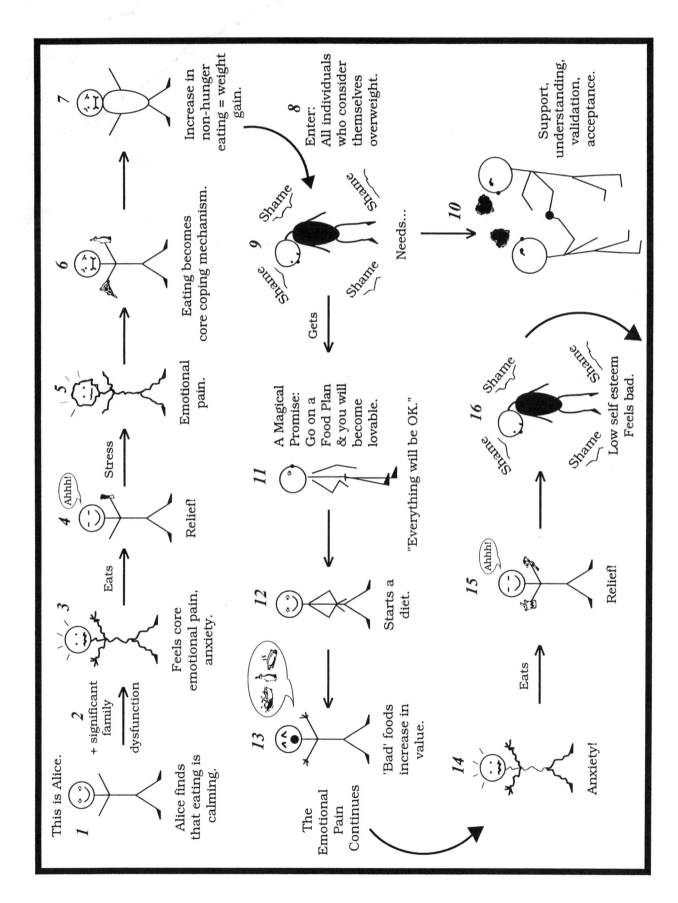

10. Alice learns that fat is bad. She believes her behavior (eating style) is what causes her to feel bad. She needs help. Help comes in one of two forms. The first form addresses the internal world: her emotions and natural internal cues.

Note to the health care provider: The healthy and most effective alternative is not to address the fat! The first alternative addresses the internal world and can occur at any time in the cycle. Healing and reconnection begin when you address distressing issues, affirm feelings, and identify behaviors in a nonjudgmental manner. Sometimes just validating a client's feelings can be healing, for example:
> "You know, I've noticed you've been eating more lately and it seems that you are eating when you are not hungry. Often that is a signal that a person is uncomfortable. I wonder if you may be uncomfortable? Or maybe sad?"

Neutralizing the behavior by communicating without moral judgment of "good" or "bad" can help the individual feel safe enough to share, for example:
> "It's normal to eat when you're not hungry. Normal eaters do it, too. However, when you do it frequently, you will probably gain weight."

Alice can learn she is not bad. In a non shaming environment, Alice can realize she does not have to lose weight to be a good person. She can start listening to her internal signals of hunger and satiety, and deal with distress in more effective ways. She can avoid getting stuck in the dieting cycle, therefore never having to obsess about food and weight. She can avoid gaining more weight. Unfortunately, this rarely occurs in our culture.

11. The second form of help addresses the outer world. Society believes fat is bad, fat is the problem. If Alice can "fix" the fat, the problem will go away.

12. Alice seeks a way to get rid of the fat. She is told to eat less fat. She feels extraordinarily hopeful when she starts the diet. She is told to divide food into "good food" and "bad food" categories. "Don't eat the 'bad' foods and you will get better." The "relief" of the diet masks her deeper distress. Temporarily, she does feel better.

13. She begins to ignore her internal signals of hunger and satiety. She also starts to obsess about foods she cannot have; a normal response to restriction. When food is forbidden, it becomes overvalued and more desired. A cookie is a cookie to a normal eater. But to a dieter, a cookie is a COOKIE! Very different.

14. Alice's distress continues unresolved.

15. She continues to eat to get relief.

16. She eats more due to built-up deprivation. She binges on forbidden foods in response to the deprivation. Why? She doesn't know why. She is told it is a lack of willpower, or she suspects she is not good enough. She is ashamed of herself and her behavior. Obviously she cannot trust herself. Her self-esteem lowers and she believes, "I'm bad."

17. She feels weak inside and says, "I need help. Another professional will help me. They tell me they have the answer."

18. Professionals do have the "answer!" A stricter diet! "A stricter diet will help me lose weight and then I'll feel better."

Figure 3-B   THE DIETING CYCLE

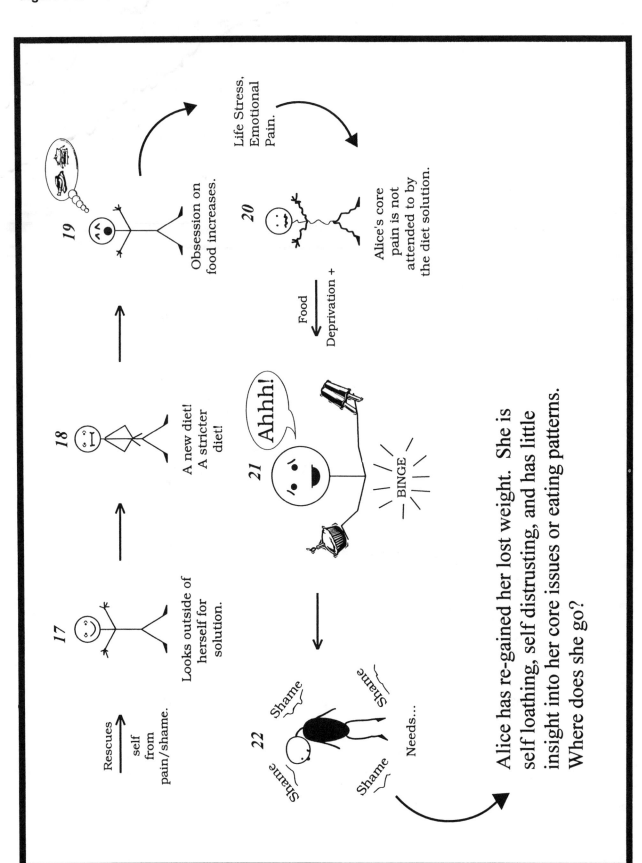

Note to the health care provider: It may be affirming to your client to point out that this repeat dieting pattern is extremely common and understandable. Individuals commonly start with a weight loss program with less restriction and then progress to stricter diets...possibly ending up at a physician-based fasting program. (This is not a comment on the effectiveness of the programs, just a comment on a dieting pattern seen in many clients.)

19. The "good" food list gets shorter, and the "bad" list gets longer. The obsession with food increases.

20.   Alice's core pain and life issues are ignored because the focus is on her food and weight, the external. Her distress is building.

21.   The combination of food obsession, deprivation, and distress become more overwhelming. Alice needs to eat more (binge eat) to get relief.

22.   Alice is becoming increasingly angry and ashamed, but hides it as she does so many other emotions.

The Process Continues
Rage builds. A wound develops. The wound is caused by years of deprivation. It hurts from being shamed by physicians, family, and friends, and from having needs and feelings ignored (notably hunger, one of the most powerful of needs). Loneliness pervades from distrust and disconnection from self as well as the isolation that results from being an "obese" person in our culture. Unfortunately, Alice has not *yet* been exposed to the first alternative: caring for the internal world. When she does receive care for her inner world she will begin to heal, to reconnect.

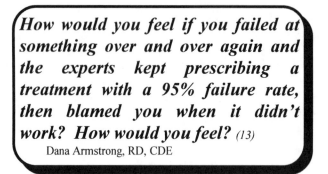

How would you feel if you failed at something over and over again and the experts kept prescribing a treatment with a 95% failure rate, then blamed you when it didn't work? How would you feel? (13)
Dana Armstrong, RD, CDE

Note to the health care provider: The wound worsens by having weight loss applauded. Imagine a client telling you, "I've lost 10 pounds in the last three weeks!" An automatic response may be, "Great, congratulations!" What is so "great" about it? Rather than applaud weight loss, ask, "Oh, how do you feel about that?" If they feel good about it, that is fine. However, sometimes this question helps the client recognize ambivalence about losing weight, or deeper feelings about living in a culture that values individuals based on appearance. It may also give them an opportunity to share past experiences where they were applauded for weight loss, but when they gained it back, felt embarrassment and shame.

SUMMARY
You must address the causes of disconnected eating (food deprivation and eating in response to emotions) in order to normalize eating, neutralize food, heal the wound, and temper the rage. Then you can work on the real issues covered up so long ago. Psychotherapy is recommended to deal with the primary issues and resultant feelings. The three facets of HungerWork detailed in the following three chapters will enable the client to:

- neutralize food (remove "good" and "bad" labels),
- reconnect with and eat in response to internal cues,
- lift deprivation,
- discern emotional needs from physical needs,
- rediscover the joy and nourishment of eating.

SELECTED RESOURCES

It's Not About Food: Healing the Obsession. Barbar Reiner Yaffee. White Seminars & Productions, P.O. Box 835, Santa Ynez, CA 93460. (800) 263-4217 (3 video tapes $225 + 9.00)
> This is a three part video seminar about women and food for professionals treating people with compulsive eating disorders and for people who are interested in their own recovery.

Tending the Soul. Francie White. White Seminars & Productions, P.O. Box 835, Santa Ynez, CA 93460. (800) 263-4217 (4 audio tapes $39.00 + 5.00 s/h)
> Live recordings from Tending the Soul workshops for professionals and nonprofessionals. Francie follows our cultural loss of soul-life with the epidemic body hatred and eating problems. Includes healing perspectives on spirituality.

The Famine Within. Video. Canada: Kandor Productions. (310) 636-8200
> A documentary outlining the origin of America's obsession with thinness. Interviews with clients with eating disorders, therapists, athletes, sociologists, feminists, anthropologists, even fashion industry moguls, are a highlight. Excellent for men and women, adolescence through adulthood.

Nourishing Wisdom: A Mind-Body Approach to Nutrition and Well-Being, David Marc. New York: Crown Publishers, Inc.; 1991.
> Marc explores an individual's relationship with food and its influence on total health, as opposed to simply analyzing the quality of food intake. The plethora of confusing nutrition messages being fed to the consumer make pleasurable eating experiences more scarce. Includes the often quoted, highly effective "Eater's Agreement." This piece establishes and entitles individuals to accept their bodies, its needs and live in accordance with such.

REFERENCES
1. Bloom C, Gitter A, Gutwill S, Kogel L, Zaphiropoulos L. *Eating Problems: A Feminist Psychoanalytic Treatment Model.* New York, NY: Basic Books; 1994.
2. Polivy J. Psychological consequences of food restriction. *J Am Diet Assoc.* 1996; 96:589-592.
3. Crawford P, Shapiro L. How obesity develops: A new look at nature and nurture - Berkeley Longitudinal Studies. *Obes & Hlth.* 1991; 3:40-41.
4. Johnson SL, Birch LL. Parents' and children's adiposity and eating style. *Peds.* 1994; 94:653-661.
5. Rose HE, Mayer J. Activity, calorie intake, fat storage and the energy balance of infants. *Peds.* 1968; 41:18-29.
6. King NL, Shifting Guidance from Outside to Within, *On the Cutting Edge.* 1995; 16: 21-24.
7. Bruce B., Wilfley D. Binge eating among the overweight population: A serious and prevalent problem. *J Am Diet Assoc.* 1996; 96:58-61.
8. Polivy J, Heatherton TF, Herman CP. Self-esteem, restraint, and eating behavior. *J of Abnormal Psych.* 1988; 97: 354-356.
9. Polivy J, Herman CP. Dieting and bingeing, a causal analysis. *Am Psych.* 1985; 40:193-201.
10. White F. "The Dieting Cycle." Original illustration. 1996. Santa Barbara, CA.
11. Anderson AD, ed. *Males with Eating Disorders.* New York, NY: Brunner/Mazel; 1990.
12. Waterhouse D. *Why Women Need Chocolate.* New York, NY: Hyperion; 1995.
13. Armstrong D. Presentation. 1994. Santa Barbara, CA.

4

HUNGER WORK: Discover Physically-Connected Eating

> *When food is stripped of its dignity, its significance, and its power, it eventually fights back, demanding our attention and tempting our all-or-nothing resolves. We will not be healthier, both psychologically and physically, about our food until we learn to love it more, not less...with a relaxed, generous, unashamed emotion (1).*

HungerWork, developed by Kratina and King, is the process by which you can help your client find the freedom to eat when hungry, quit when satisfied, and do so, free of negative self-talk and critical judgment. It involves rediscovering the contentment that comes from nourishing, joyful eating. The next three chapters are dedicated to the three facets of HungerWork.

- Discover physically-connected eating
  - a. Neutralize food
  - b. Identify and interpret hunger and satiety cues
- Heal disconnected eating: Identify and decode eating experiences
- Promote joyful and healthful eating

Each of these facets of HungerWork addresses an aspect where disconnection may occur between a person's food and body relationship. Physically-connected eating results from moving through all three facets of HungerWork. It is characterized by:

- Eating when hungry and stopping when full or satisfied.
- Eating enough to be sustained to the next meal or snack, arriving at the preferred hunger level.
- Choosing foods that are varied, wholesome, satisfying, and health enhancing.
- Tempering choices with nutrition knowledge and scientific facts.
- Living free of worry, obsession or preoccupation with food, the body, and eating.

NEUTRALIZE FOOD: THE FIRST STEP IN DISCOVERING PHYSICALLY-CONNECTED EATING
Perhaps the most disturbing, and disheartening, aspect of the current food paranoia is that it seems driven far more by a fear of death than by a love of life. It is possible to become so engaged in the business of fleeing illness and decay that one forgets how to truly and fully live--or forgets that one point of living is to enjoy (1).

It is clear the quality and quantity of foods a person eats impact his or her health and sense of well-being. For example: some foods are more nutrient-dense than others (peaches are a richer source of potassium than iceberg lettuce), or excesses of saturated fats can raise blood cholesterol levels in predisposed individuals. In an effort to communicate this knowledge in a simplified manner to the public it seems natural to categorize foods as "good" or "bad." Some of the negative consequences of this division of foods now are becoming more apparent. An individual uses the authorities' moralized labeling of foods to help control his or her food intake. This is an attempt to gain control over food and behaviors that could control them or have controlled them in the past. The cacophony of moralized messages may sound something like this:

> [neu tral] adjective. Neither positive nor negative (2).

"But fat *is* bad, isn't it?"
"Eliminate the fat from your diet."
"Fat makes you fat."
"Eat fat-free cake and cookies instead."
"Isn't frozen yogurt healthier?"
"The polyunsaturated fat is good for you, but the saturated fat may clog your heart and arteries and cause a heart attack. Stay away from it."
"As soon as I cut out fat, the next thing I hear is starches make you fat."

> **"Food guilt" is rampant in our culture and Americans eat every day. What does that say about our mental health?** Karin Kratina, MA, RD

Some people hear these messages and say, "Well, maybe I will cut *some* fat out by skipping the butter tonight." Others, ostensibly seeking greater control, take this further and conclude, "I shouldn't eat that...I must cut out *all* fat...Fat is so bad for me...It's gross and disgusting (3)." As these thoughts intensify, a fear of food develops.

Fear-Based Food Choices

An individual begins to select food based on fear in the quest for control of weight, eating behaviors, or health. Media, health care providers, and educators promulgate these fears. Some nutrition messages inadvertently perpetuate these fears in an effort to increase awareness and prompt behavior changes (social marketing). For example, a dietitian might say, "Did you know there are four teaspoons of fat in that cheese?" Although the intent is to increase awareness, these messages become internalized and most food selection eventually is based on these fears. "Bad food" lists get longer, and avoiding these foods becomes paramount. Furthermore, these individuals may be admired by others for their discipline. This provides additional reinforcement for their fear-based eating style.

Avoidance May Lead to Obsession

What is the problem with food fears or labeling? Most individuals think if a food is labeled "bad" it will be avoided. *Unfortunately, when individuals purposely avoid something, they tend to think about it more.* This may be easier to understand away from the emotionally charged arena of food.

For example, consider Barbara, who hates to fly. When a trip is being planned, she immediately begins to obsess about transportation. "Will I have to fly? Is there another way to get there? Can I cancel my trip? Can I get a tranquilizer?" Adrienne on the other hand, sees flying as a way to get from point A to point B. She doesn't love it, nor does she hate it. Sometimes it's fun, but always it's a necessity. Flying for her is a neutral activity. Who thinks about flying more often? In trying to avoid it,

Barbara actually thinks about it more. The same thing happens with food. The more effort put into avoiding a food, the more important it becomes; the more often it is thought about (3).

Shutting Down Exploration

This way of looking at food--coldly, with distance and distrust becomes self-perpetuating. Our current situation is not going to lead to furthering the enjoyment and experience of food. And that's a real problem, because the experience and acknowledgment of food brings more self-awareness, and self-awareness will bring self-control (1).

The implications of the good/bad, legal/illegal food paradigm run deeper than the labeling alone. When a food is labeled, the individual's exploration, discovery, and natural feedback process is suppressed. Exploration and discovery involve asking such questions as, "Do I like the way this food feels in my body? Am I comfortable with the fullness level? Do I feel energized? How long will the food sustain me?" Instead of being open to the natural feedback, the individual predetermines a "good" or "bad" outcome based on which list ("good" or "bad") the food is on. In reality, food's *impact* on health, weight, and well-being can be viewed as positive or negative, but these results are influenced by the frequency, amount, and most importantly, the individual's physical and psychological status. Food, itself, is neutral.   The next four examples show clients making cognitive or emotional decisions about food and the "expected" outcome, rather than being open to the actual outcome:

1. Sarah knows she has a long night of studying ahead so she purchases snack foods to help her stay awake in the late hours. She is caught in the dilemma of wanting to snack, but trying to be "good." She settles on red licorice, fat-free. She begins snacking on the licorice and hopes it won't "make her fat." By midnight she has eaten 10 sticks. She worries about weight gain from eating the licorice. First thing in the morning she weighs. Her weight is the same as the day before. She cannot figure it out. She obsesses about her weight the rest of the day, weighing herself at least four more times. By the end of the day, after consuming a minimal amount of food and multiple cans of diet soda, Sarah sees the scale register three additional pounds. She was "good" all day, so the weight gain must be from the licorice the night before. It finally caught up with her, she thinks.

Notice how Sarah expected to gain weight based upon eating the licorice, a decided "bad" food. When she did not gain as expected, she concluded her body was not responding as it should. When her weight did go up from the fluid intake, she placed the blame on the licorice. Discovering and gently challenging Sarah's belief system about weight and weight shifts, along with what foods Sarah thinks are "bad" or "good" will be helpful. *Affirming that eating a wide variety of foods, even the so called "bad" foods, when she is hungry and stopping when she is comfortably full or satisfied will not change her weight. These are fundamental concepts she will need to hear many times as she rebuilds trust in her body and food.*

2. In a session with his nutrition therapist Matthew states, "At noon I ate a huge garden salad with fat-free dressing, one piece of the crusty French bread, no butter, and a couple glasses of iced tea with lemon. It was a lot of food. I felt stuffed. I thought I was eating right. I don't see how I could possibly be hungry at 4:00 p.m."

Notice in this example how labeling food "good" or "bad" confuses the client's interpretation of their internal cues. Matthew can begin to trust his body cues if he is affirmed that although his lunch choices were health enhancing, based on the caloric intake, it would be normal to need "refueling" within a 1-2 hour time frame. Can he look back to 1:30-2:00 in the afternoon and recall feeling hunger begin to build? If Matthew prefers to postpone hunger for more than a couple of hours, guide him in exploring the types of foods and quantities of each (proteins, fat, carbohydrates, and fiber) that will elicit this response.

3. Eight year old Jamie eats 15 homemade chocolate chip cookies then complains her stomach hurts. Jamie's mother responds with, "Eating that many cookies is bad for you. You should have known better.

No wonder your stomach hurts." The message is, "That was a bad thing to do." This may then be interpreted as "I am bad for doing that," particularly with children (4). The resulting negative feelings often cause a person to eat even more cookies.

Consider if the mother instead said, "Yes, your stomach is hurting. That's natural when you put many cookies into it." This message is, "It's natural for my stomach to hurt with this many cookies." Jamie is affirmed. Since there was no "bad" or guilt, she is free, and empowered, to decide if she again wants to eat so much her stomach hurts. She probably won't.

4. A client, Elinor, recently reported she had eaten eggplant rotini and said, "That's really bad, isn't it?" The counselor said, "What do you mean?" Elinor replied, "Well, it's bad for you, it's fried and full of cheese. It's full of fat and it's gross. It's bad, right?" The counselor told her "No." Elinor got angry saying, "I shouldn't be eating these kinds of foods. I'm too fat anyway. Of course it's bad." Then the counselor asked how her body felt after she ate it. As she paused to think about the question, it was apparent this was an unfamiliar perspective. Finally, she said, "I felt gross, and it was because I ate such bad food." The counselor processed this and finally asked if she felt "gross" because she ate *more than her body needed* (not "too much," a moralizing term). After some resistance, Elinor realized she had become uncomfortably full, and that was what had made her uncomfortable.

> *Moralizing gives food the power to make individuals feel good and to feel bad about themselves. This moralization is born in a social context (and learned very early in life) from the messages in the environment (5).*

These types of situations are excellent opportunities to help clients discover:
- the tastes of food,
- the way food feels in their body,
- the resulting energy level from eating food,
- the duration of satiety, fullness, and sustenance...all without judgment.

STRATEGIES AND TECHNIQUES TO NEUTRALIZE FOOD

But, the true cure for our dietary sins may lie in an almost opposite direction to that prescribed by the nutrition experts--not in claiming more control, but less; not in taking power away from food, but giving it back; not in fear of death, but in love of life. Somewhere in the ancient love of food and its rituals lies rationality and reverence for natural things and a balanced sense of how much is too much--colored by scientific knowledge, but not ruled by it (1).

Following are strategies and techniques you can use to help clients move beyond "good food, bad food" labels:

1. Rephrase terms that have moral overtones or make value judgments.

Moralized/Judgmental		Nonjudgmental
"You did well this week."	*becomes...*	"I'm happy you got in all your protein. Could you tell me about it?"
"Too much fat is bad for you."	*becomes...*	"Sometimes when people eat a high fat diet, they feel sluggish, is that happening for you?"
"My blood glucose is high because I cheated by eating pie."	*becomes...*	"I notice my blood glucose elevates when I eat a piece of pie before bed."

2. View individual foods in relation to daily intake. Ask the client to name a "healthy" food. They may reply, "Broccoli." Ask them to imagine eating only broccoli for one day. Could the broccoli be considered a health enhancing food in this context? Since broccoli cannot provide all the nutrients their body needs, it cannot be considered a health enhancing food when eaten in this way. Although this is an extreme example, you can use this type of approach to explore clients' belief systems with various foods. This type of reframing can help clients become more flexible in their food choices and less judgmental of those choices.

3. Appreciate the social context of eating. Lisa is playing cards with her son who is eating chips and salsa. This is what Lisa really wants, but, to be "good" she decides to munch on carrots. She is trying to connect with her son, but finds she is distracted by her desire for the chips and the energy she is devoting to stay away from them. She is not enjoying the carrots either. Lisa obsesses more about the chips because she believes they are "bad" and because she will not allow herself to eat them. How "healthy" are those carrots? If Lisa and her counselor explore her experience, they may discover when she force feeds (the carrots) and restricts (the chips) there is little enjoyment and less energy to devote to the special moments in her life.

4. Put on "eating disorder" glasses before reading anything about food, eating, or weight. In all types of media, clients regularly read headlines such as, "How to Get Rid of Excess Fat,"... "Eat Less Fat in Your Diet." Depending upon the individual's perspective, these messages can be very harmful. Filtering these messages through the "eyes" of someone with eating problems can help prevent the development of harmful eating practices. Concerning the above message, someone with disordered eating probably will not ask, "Less fat than what?" They will assume the least amount of fat intake is the best. You can help the client discern the realistic, health enhancing messages from the health detracting claims.

5. Avoid foods if they produce a negative outcome. If Alex gets heartburn when he eats French fries, he may choose to avoid them or eat smaller amounts. This choice is based on the outcome, not because French fries are good or bad. Working with clients and eating problems is challenging--clients often present/ arrive with a long list of "undesirable" foods. You may need to explore the client's relationship with each food to determine why the food is undesirable. Does it cause heartburn because of the quantity eaten? Is the food not "safe"? ("Safe" foods are foods the client is comfortable eating without worry, guilt, fear, or tendency to binge eat.) Do they binge on the food? Is it a forbidden food? Is the food not "allowed"? Is the food "bad"? What other beliefs does this client have about the food? Explore with questions such as these to help clients remove foods from the "bad" list and view them as neutral.

6. Evaluate fuel put into the body without judgment. Tom owns two cars; a diesel station wagon and a weekend sports car. Each time he buys gas, Tom has a choice in fuel. Tom's decision is not based on good or bad fuel, but what would work best in each car. In the station wagon he is careful to use only diesel fuel, having been warned non-diesel fuel could damage the engine. In the same way, when he wants to drive his sports car through the mountains on a Sunday afternoon, he can choose from several different grades of gasoline. Tom's appreciation for his sports car prompted him to consult the owner's manual to determine the best gas for performance, fuel efficiency, and longevity. Tom tried a lower octane fuel to save a few dollars. However, he noticed the car started to knock and ping. Tom realized he needed quality fuel so the sports car would run its best and provide the most fun. Tom does not criticize himself for trying lower octane fuel, but listens to his car's feedback and chooses higher octane fuel. The human body provides similar feedback.

It is important to model for your clients being open and free of judgment when they are experimenting with food and listening to their bodies' feedback. Fear, confusion, misunderstanding, and dissatisfaction in their eating experiences needs to be recognized and explored. Working with your clients in this subjective realm frees them to develop a satisfying, health enhancing relationship with food.

IDENTIFY AND INTERPRET HUNGER AND SATIETY CUES:
THE SECOND STEP TO DISCOVER PHYSICALLY-CONNECTED EATING

The Science of Hunger and Satiety

> *...increasing consumption of carbohydrate at the expense of fat could cause hunger to return sooner because of decreased secretion of cholecystokinin. To put it another way, food intake is undoubtedly regulated by a variety of cues, one of which may be the amount of fat in our diet. When we reduce fat intake, we may be giving up one of the cues that tells us when we have had enough to eat* (6).

For many health care providers, education and training did not extensively discuss the concept of regulating food and nutrient intake by internal cues, such as hunger, satiety, appetite, and fullness. Perhaps the only significant reference to hunger in training was as a critical social issue.

These internal cues are not just about perceiving an empty or full feeling in the stomach area. They are important components in a partially understood, complex mix of psychological and physiological factors all relating to satisfaction (7). Research has attempted to identify what prompts individuals to start and stop eating, and explain why they make the food choices they do. Listening to clients share their experiences reveals their perception and interpretation of hunger and its associated internal cues. The bottom line is, people primarily make food choices based upon taste and satisfaction (8).

Some studies show that "dietary fat does not significantly enhance satiety in obese individuals (9,10)." Another study demonstrates that the elderly may be at risk for many nutrition-related acute or chronic illnesses as they have difficulty perceiving their hunger and fullness cues (11). Allred (6) suggests that the U.S. trend toward reduction of dietary fat intake may be correlated to its increase in body fat.

Perhaps the most significant and relevant research to the nondiet approach is on restrained eaters. Studies show that a history of restrained eating (dieting) interferes with an individual's ability to self-regulate food intake using hunger and fullness cues. There is a resultant increased tendency to binge eat, and/ or continue eating when full. Whether restriction is voluntary or involuntary, there are psychological side effects such as: food preoccupation, emotional lability, diminished tolerance of emotions, especially ego-related, and heightened distractibility (12).

Combining the client's experience with research can help explain why people in the U.S. are not eating in accordance with their internal cues. At any one time 46 million people in the U.S. are dieting (13). An astonishing 81% of 10 year old girls (middle class) are afraid of being fat (14). In a study of 1,268 adolescent females, 52% began dieting before age 14 (15). The U.S. population is clearly in a crisis about food, weight, and health. On a deeper level, the crisis is about acknowledging needs and entitlement to satisfying them. *Moving away from diets allows individuals to begin experiencing less stress, dissatisfaction, and harm in response to their need to eat.*

Strategies and Techniques to Reconnect with Hunger and Satiety
Hunger is one of the first intense, urgent, repetitive, internal experiences.
If hunger is quickly followed by satisfaction, the infant learns that hunger is manageable (16).

The following terms are used in the characterization of physically-connected eating (2):

Hunger--the state of discomfort or weakness caused by lack of food.
Appetite--a desire for food or drink.
Fullness--having had ample food or drink.
Satisfaction/Satiety--having satisfied the appetite or desire.

Discerning physical cues of hunger and satiety from cognitive, behavioral, or emotional cues is a challenging and rewarding aspect of HungerWork. As clients move to physically-connected eating they learn to determine:

- when and what to eat by listening to internal signals of hunger and appetite;
- how much food to eat by listening to the body's signals of satiety and fullness;
- when food is wanted for reasons other than physical hunger, and determine the desired course of action. (Emotions can cue eating as can memories, celebrations, habits and routines.)
- how to temper the above with a relaxed interpretation of what science reports is health enhancing.

When the client can consistently make physically-connected food choices, the result is repeatedly feeling energized and nourished by the chosen foods. This adds to the anticipation and enjoyment of the eating experience. You can use the following five strategies and techniques to teach your clients how to identify, interpret, and trust internal cues of hunger, fullness, appetite, and satiety.

1. Explore the client's perception of physical hunger. When you ask clients how hungry they are, often the responses are nebulous:
"Oh, I don't know. I could eat something, I guess."
"I've been busy all day, so I haven't gotten hungry."
"It's not time to eat (as they glance at the clock)."
These answers may indicate clients either do not notice hunger unless it is quite intense or they are unfamiliar with how hunger progresses throughout the day. They may be unfamiliar or uncomfortable talking about hunger. In this discussion it is important that you are clearly nonjudgmental from the start. The following questions are helpful when exploring hunger, appetite, fullness, and satiety with clients:
How do you know when you are hungry?
Can you touch the part(s) of your body where you feel hunger? Fullness?
Do you experience different types of hunger? More gradual onset versus urgent?
Does your hunger vary from day to day?
How do you know when you are full? Satisfied? What's the difference?
Have you ever felt full, but not satisfied? Have you ever felt satisfied, but not full?

How do you decide when to start eating and stop eating?

How do you feel about yourself/food/body when you are hungry/full/satisfied?

What happens to your hunger if you do not eat right away?

Is there an intensity of hunger or fullness that is uncomfortable? Why is that?

Is your desire for food or the taste of food affected by your hunger or fullness level?

How often do you eat your favorite foods? Is that your preference?

Do you feel differently about your body when you are hungry? Full?

Do you feel fat when you are full? Thin when you feel hungry?

Would your *eating* style be different from what it is now if *food* did not impact your weight or
your health? (You also can insert *exercise* or *physical activity*.)

When was the last time you ate and felt satisfied?

What do you typically do if you are eating and realize the food is not enjoyable?

2. Quantify and monitor physical cues using the Hunger Scale. After discussing hunger and fullness using some of the above questions, you can introduce the Hunger Scale on the Food Journal, Figure 4-A. In this scale 0 represents empty, 5 represents neutral, and 10 represents stuffed. The following brief analogy is helpful:

"Imagine you are a car. When your gas tank is completely empty this registers as a 0. When the tank is 'topped off' you are at 10. Five is neutral, neither full nor empty, halfway."

Although this analogy describes absolute emptiness and fullness, the Hunger Scale is meant to be subjective. It is the client's interpretation of a 2 versus 3 or 7 versus 8 that is the standard. Refrain from defining all the numbers for them other than 0,5,10. Use open-ended questions to help the client discern and communicate the numbers. Encourage self-discovery and self-acceptance by being open to subjectivity. Let your client know you are interested in learning about them. Defining numbers on the Hunger Scale allows them to develop a "language" for communicating thoughts, feelings, and experiences related to their physical cues.

In the accompanying food journal, notice there are no specific time slots for meals, since it is normal to vary eating patterns. The absence of time slots discourages the notion that there are "right" or "wrong" times to eat.

Many clients have difficulty discerning degrees of hunger initially, especially clients with extensive dieting histories. Furthermore, most find that being attentive to physical cues is awkward and, for some, extremely uncomfortable. You can reinforce the nonjudgmental environment by assuring clients that many people feel uncertain or lack confidence in reading internal cues. Explain that this is a process of exploration and discovery; there are no right or wrong answers. One of the most important characteristics you can demonstrate is speaking gently and patiently with clients, so they in turn can do this for themselves.

Getting in touch with hunger may begin by suggesting the client "check in and take a reading" hourly or when eating. Recording hunger and fullness levels frequently (perhaps hourly) in the journal will help them recognize subtle changes as hunger or fullness intensify (17).

Note: Have clients fill in square that reflects their present status. If they are eating or drinking, they continue to fill in squares up to the square that reflects their fullness at the end of the eating experience.

Occasionally, clients will not be able to perceive any hunger or fullness cues. Some of the more common barriers to recognizing these cues follow:

- being afraid their needs are too great to be met, and subsequently deny them;
- feeling undeserving of having needs met before they meet someone (everyone) else's;

continued on page 52

Figure 4-A FOOD JOURNAL with HUNGER SCALE and FEELINGS JOURNAL

FOOD JOURNAL

NAME: _____

DATE: _____

DAY: M T W Th F Sa Su

TODAY'S GOAL AND/OR AFFIRMATION: _____

TIME	FOOD AND QUANTITY	DP	B/MP	F/V	G	O	HUNGER SCALE 0 1 2 3 4 5 6 7 8 9 10	MOOD, THOUGHTS AND/OR FEELINGS
TOTALS								
RECOMMENDED								

0 = Empty 5 = Neutral 10 = Stuffed

Graph hunger level from start to end of meal

EXERCISE: _____

DP = Dairy Protein
B/MP = Bean / Meat Protein
F/V = Fruit / Vegetable
G = Grain
O = Others

© Copyright 1993 Karin Kratina MA, RD / Reflective Image, Inc., Publishers 1993

- remembering painful memories (i.e. physical or sexual abuse, trauma, or uncomfortable sensations) when they identify internal cues;
- being inattentive throughout the eating experience, thereby not noticing fullness;
- being distracted by the eating process itself;
- obsessing about what they did or did not consume, and the consequences.

If clients have trouble identifying hunger, ask them to postpone a meal one hour or two prior to their session. Allow them a few moments to "check in and take a reading" of their hunger level. If they are unsure of the number, discuss what sensations they are feeling. Using a meal clients bring to the session (make sure it is an ample amount), invite them to begin eating. Encourage a slow, relaxed pace while discussing the physical changes they notice as the food is being digested. Help the client put their experiences into words and begin placing the degree of fullness on the 0-10 Hunger Scale. Some clients may find it helpful if you eat your meal as they eat theirs. Others will find this distracting or divert attention off themselves onto you.

It is possible an individual may have organic problems that require medical assessment or psychological issues that require more intensive psychotherapeutic intervention. A psychiatrist, aware of hunger and satiety issues, may be able to assess these types of situations.

SUSAN'S FOOD JOURNAL

Figure 4-B is Susan's first attempt at tracking her hunger and fullness. Readings may appear inconsistent and somewhat inaccurate. (Usually, readings are somewhat inconsistent for the first few weeks until the client gains more experience gauging cues.) Notice Susan has some wide swings (2-9) and narrow (3-6), (5 to 5). These may be actual readings or just lack of experience. Asking her to describe sensations she feels at a 9 and compare to a 6, or a 10 will help her fine tune her definitions of the varying intensities.

Reiterate to Susan, "This is an entirely different way to pay attention to yourself. After a variety of experiences, you will be more confident identifying the subtle differences between a 3, 4, and 5. This scale will provide insights for our work together and it will prove invaluable to you over your lifetime. Let's be patient with the process, O.K.?"

Note: If clients are restricting (eating less than approximately 1,300 calories per day), are binge eating and purging, or are in exceptional emotional distress, they may not be able to track hunger and fullness accurately because their cues may be skewed. Let them know that they may not experience common hunger cues because the restriction of calories is more serious than just a matter of "refueling." Additionally, these clients may have extraordinary fears and anxieties about identifying, interpreting and responding to their hunger and fullness cues.

These clients may, however, be able to identify cues that are more characteristic of the side effects of starvation identified in the Keyes study "The Biology of Starvation" (18). These include: dizziness, cold sensitivity, food preoccupation, decreased concentration, extreme weakness, tiredness, depression, anxiety, isolating behavior, mood swings, and sleep disturbances. Until the client can eat in a sound manner, monitor these symptoms as one sign of progress. Clients can record them on the right hand side of the food/feelings journal (Moods, Thoughts, and/or Feelings).

In contrast, clients engaged in a binge eating style (such as Binge Eating Disorder or Night Eating Syndrome) may have reliable cues. Clients with anorexia nervosa who had a sound eating style in recovery, but then recycle, are often able to do HungerWork. One of the most traumatic experiences in recovery for some clients with anorexia seems to be encountering intense hunger sensations that make it virtually impossible to tolerate restricting their food and starving themselves again.

3. Experiment with the Meal Mix.
   Although the types of carbohydrates or fats in foods may affect hunger and food intake within and between meals, more experiments are required to determine effects on daily energy intake (19).

Figure 4-B   SUSAN'S FOOD JOURNAL

FOOD JOURNAL

NAME: Susan
DATE: 6/25/96
DAY: M (T) W Th F Sa Su

TODAY'S GOAL AND/OR AFFIRMATION: Can pay closer attention to my body's cues.

TIME	FOOD AND QUANTITY	DP	B/MP	F/V	G	O	HUNGER SCALE (0 1 2 3 4 5 6 7 8 9 10)	MOOD, THOUGHTS AND/OR FEELINGS
6:30	English muffin, margarine, orange juice (large)							Wasn't very hungry. Felt very full, maybe from orange juice.
8:30	Bran muffin, Coffee, black (2)							Office meeting. Saw the muffin and got hungry.
12:30	Chicken tostada, Iced tea, chips & salsa							Ate all my meal because I was starving! Got too full. Could've been ok with less.
3:30	Skittles (pack)							Wanted something sweet.
6:30	Dinner salad at restaurant, French bread (3 slices) w/ butter, Iced tea.							Didn't feel hungry or full. Ate too much bread.
TOTALS								
RECOMMENDED								

DP = Dairy Protein
B/MP = Bean / Meat Protein
F/V = Fruit / Vegetable
G = Grain
O = Others

0 = Empty
5 = Neutral
10 = Stuffed

Graph hunger level from start to end of meal

EXERCISE:

© Copyright 1993 Karin Kratina MA, RD / Reflective Image, Inc., Publishers 1993

Figure 4-C ALEXIS' FOOD JOURNAL

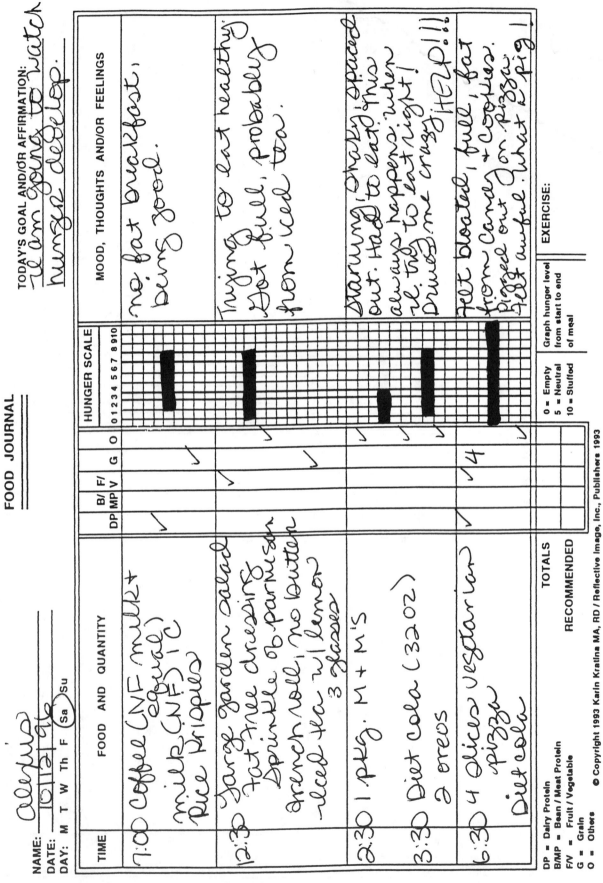

FOOD JOURNAL

NAME: Alexis
DATE: 10/12/96
DAY: M T W Th F (Sa) Su

TODAY'S GOAL AND/OR AFFIRMATION:
I am going to watch hunger develop.

TIME	FOOD AND QUANTITY	DP	B/MP	F/V	G	O	HUNGER SCALE 0 1 2 3 4 5 6 7 8 9 10	MOOD, THOUGHTS AND/OR FEELINGS
7:00	Coffee (NF milk + equal) milk (NF) 1C Rice Krispies	✓			✓	✓		no fat breakfast, being good.
12:30	large garden salad fat free dressing sprinkle of parmesan french roll, no butter iced tea w/ lemon 3 grapes			✓	✓	✓		Trying to eat healthy. Not full, probably from iced tea.
3:30	1 pkg. M + M's					✓		Starving, shaky, spaced out. Had to eat. This always happens when I try to eat right! Drives me crazy. HELP!!!
3:30	Diet Cola (32 oz) 2 oreos					✓		
6:30	4 slices vegetarian pizza Diet cola	✓			✓4	✓		Felt bloated, full, fat from candy + cookies. Pigged out on pizza. Felt awful. What a pig!
	TOTALS							EXERCISE:
	RECOMMENDED							

Graph hunger level from start to end of meal

0 = Empty
5 = Neutral
10 = Stuffed

DP = Dairy Protein
B/MP = Bean / Meat Protein
F/V = Fruit / Vegetable
G = Grain
O = Other

© Copyright 1993 Karin Kratina MA, RD / Reflective Image, Inc., Publishers 1993

The Hunger Scale can be used to work in the objective realm; discovering optimal "meal mix," that is, the proportion of protein, fat, and carbohydrate desired and needed by the client. (Meal mix also considers simple and complex carbohydrates, fiber, caffeine, alcohol, artificial sweeteners, and medications.) Clients begin to notice some meals and snacks postpone hunger longer than others. This is an opportunity for the nutrition professional to interpret or affirm these responses. (Meal mix is discussed again in chapter 6.)

In the food/feelings journal for Alexis, Figure 4-C, notice the hunger comes on suddenly following a lunch relatively high in carbohydrates and low in fat and protein. She attempts to "rescue" herself by eating candy at 2:30 p.m. to bring her glucose level back up and abate the hunger. She thinks this should last her, after all, candy is "so fattening." It did not fill her, though. She is driven to eat only one hour later (3:30 p.m.) due to hunger, low blood glucose sensations (exacerbated by caffeine intake from coffee, iced tea, and diet cola) (20), and lack of satiation from previous foods that day. By the time she gets home from work, Alexis is feeling hungry, unsatisfied, guilty, and defeated. She has tried countless times to eat "right" and she feels "starving, shaky, and spacey" every time. She finally drops her defenses and overeats pizza to get rid of hunger, to get free of restriction, and to get over the "inevitable binge."

With guidance from her health care provider, Alexis will probably discover she needs protein and some fat at lunch in order to be sustained throughout the afternoon and experience a more gradual progression of hunger rather than a "crash."

Expect variations in meal mix preferences from one client to another. For example, some clients may find fruit is an adequate breakfast food. Others may need a certain amount of fat in a meal to feel satisfied. Still others feel energized and sustained if they include foods high in protein for breakfast. Clients will discover for themselves the effect food has on their energy, appetite, satiety, fullness, subsequent hunger, moods, medical measures (such as blood glucose values), and sense of well-being. It is normal and health enhancing for total caloric intake, nutrient requirements, and meal mix to vary from day to day.

4. Examine distorted perceptions of hunger using the Hunger Scale. The Hunger Scale can help identify distortions in perceptions of hunger or fullness. For instance, a client reports eating two slices of toast and indicates she went from 2 to 9 on the Hunger Scale. Since this is not a typical response to two pieces of toast, one could assume her perception was distorted. Explore this response with questions such as:

What did it feel like to be a 9 here?
Is this 9 the same or different from other times you've been a 9?
What fullness level do you reach if you eat more than two pieces of toast?

Clients with disordered eating often use the tightness of clothes around the abdomen or the sensation of a bloated belly to determine fullness. Additionally, they may create a false sensation of fullness by engaging in negative self-talk, exaggerating the amount of calories consumed, or eating a food they believe is "bad" or associated with binge eating. The right hand side of the food/feelings journal provides clients an opportunity to write what they say to themselves (thoughts and feelings) about their hunger and fullness.

Restrained eaters have extensive experience tuning out hunger signals. Hunger may only be apparent to them when it is unavoidable (levels 0-2), and overeating or binge eating frequently results (levels 9 or 10). Often, when clients learn to get in touch with and respond to hunger at levels 3 and 4, they are less likely to overeat.

5. Enhance the usefulness of food journals. Use the following strategies to make food journals more effective:

- Invite clients to read their journals out loud in a session. This can enhance their awareness of judgmental, self-critical thinking, and can expose their fears of the health care provider's response. This provides an opportunity to begin transforming their self-talk and self-image. It also lays a vital foundation for a self-regulated eating style, free of judgment and criticism.

- Physical activity may enhance clients' perceptions of hunger and fullness. For example when they are active they may find it easier to discern between a 2 and a 4 on the Hunger Scale. Increased caloric expenditure during the activity often increases the caloric requirement. Many clients find they are more attuned to other cues as well, such as thirst, muscle tension or relaxation, and energy or fatigue as a result of being physically active.

- Guide clients into discovering the need and value of a food journal. Inform clients they are the "data gatherers" or the "fact finders." Sometimes clients suggest recording key information when presented with the following analogy: Pretend there is a videographer shadowing you all day long. He is taping "A Day in the Life of ____." Often a client will respond, "I can't remember everything like a video camera can. Would it be helpful if I wrote some of these findings down?" Sometimes, rather than furnishing a journal form to clients, they may feel inspired to create their own journals. This demonstrates motivation, self-initiative, and internal direction.

- When the session is nearing the end, make certain clients can explain exactly what they will be recording. It must seem reasonable to them, and to you, or else they are setting up for failure. If they are offering to do more than is possible in one week, explore this, and reset goals. Setting reasonable goals is critical. You must realize the goal may need to be quite simple, for example asking a client to initiate eating at a 4 rather than a 5 once this week, may be an appropriate challenge.

These treatment strategies can also be useful as you help clients discern physical hunger from emotional needs. You and your client can explore the identified feelings and possibly discover alternative coping strategies that do not use food and more directly address the feelings. (These feelings may need to be processed with a mental health professional.) Chapter 8 on counseling skills explores techniques further.

STRATEGIES AND TECHNIQUES

Any of the following treatment techniques can be used with clients in a session. Clients may gain the most from "hands on" guidance and encouragement.

Normalizing Eating Patterns Using the Hunger Scale

Tracking the Hunger Scale on a food/feelings journal can be extremely useful for identifying and resolving disconnected eating. Discover with clients what physical hunger and fullness levels they prefer. Often, their eating behaviors parallel their feelings. Work with clients to enable them to eventually stay between 3 and 7 or 8. Following are common disordered eating patterns, possible accompanying emotional patterns, and treatment strategies that may be helpful:

Case Study (Figure 4-D)

Sally swings between 1 and 9 or 10 and interprets her eating as out of control. She may have accompanying emotions that are out of control. Sometimes she is unable to provide food for herself when she needs to eat, or find comfort when she has needs or feelings to express. She may feel she does not deserve to eat unless extremely hungry, and then when she does eat, feels like she overeats.

Treatment strategy: Sally can try eating a meal when at level 2 on the 0-10 Hunger Scale and process this experience. Explore why she does not take time to eat during the day. Discuss how she uses caffeine for energy, to suppress appetite, or to distract her from feelings. Strategize with Sally how to take time to eat during the day and how to make food available that she likes. What would that entail? How does she feel about the idea? Eventually move toward eating between levels 3 and 7 or 8.

Figure 4-D SALLY'S FOOD JOURNAL

FOOD JOURNAL

NAME: SALLY
DATE: 8/24/96
DAY: M T W Th (F) Sa Su

TODAY'S GOAL AND/OR AFFIRMATION: TRY NOT TO GET SO HUNGRY. EAT SOONER!

TIME	FOOD AND QUANTITY	DP	MP	B/F/V	G	O	HUNGER SCALE (0 1 2 3 4 5 6 7 8 9 10)	MOOD, THOUGHTS AND/OR FEELINGS
9:00	CAPPUCINO							NOT HUNGRY, REALLY. VERY STRESSFUL MEETING, POTENTIAL CLIENTS.
10:30	BAGELS(2) WITH CREAM CHEESE, DONUT, COFFEE							BOSS MADE ME LOOK STUPID. I'LL TALK TO HIM MONDAY. I WAS STARVING, THEN ATE TOO MUCH.
12:30	SKIPPED LUNCH							HAD TO REWORK PROJECT FOR POTENTIAL CLIENTS...STILL UPSET. SKIPPED LUNCH TO WORK. DIDN'T WANT TO EAT ANYWAY! BLAH!
4:30	DIET COLA (2)							FLYING OUT THE DOOR TO POST OFFICE BY 5 PM. HORRIBLE STRESSFUL DAY. WHAT'S NEW? CAN'T WAIT TO GET HOME AND EAT!
6:30	CHINESE FOOD							FINALLY ATE. TOTALLY EXHAUSTED. HAD TO GET FULL...HAD TO I KNOW I SHOULDN'T THOUGH.
10:30	NOTHING. TOO FULL							
TOTALS								
RECOMMENDED								

Graph hunger level from start to end of meal
0 = Empty
5 = Neutral
10 = Stuffed

EXERCISE:

DP = Dairy Protein
B/MP = Bean / Meat Protein
F/V = Fruit / Vegetable
G = Grain
O = Others

© Copyright 1993 Karin Kratina MA, RD / Reflective Image, Inc., Publishers 1993

Figure 4-E   RITA'S FOOD JOURNAL

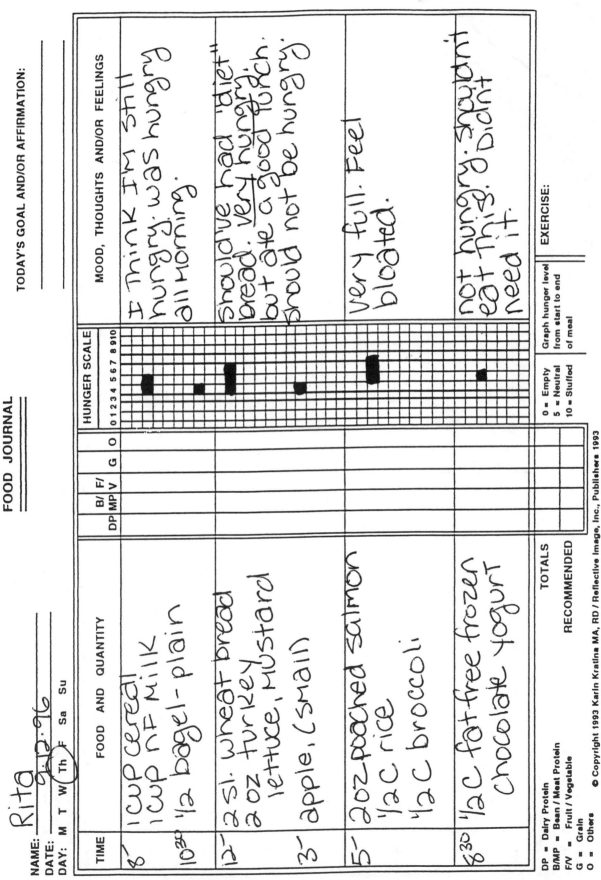

Case Study (Figure 4-E)

Rita stays between 4 and 6 on the scale. She is afraid to venture into more intense physical feelings of hunger and fullness and may subsequently keep her emotions in tight control as well. She believes a slight degree of hunger is frightening and fullness means failure. Rita is a veteran dieter and weighs and measures her food. She feels more in control of food and her feelings if she maintains this eating pattern.

Treatment strategy: In a structured, supportive environment, such as in a session, have Rita eat to level 7 on the scale and process this experience. Work toward increased flexibility and comfort, eating between levels 3 and 8. As Rita gains awareness and trust in her internal cues, move her away from weighing and measuring her food. Restrained eaters, may need to eat at a 4 or 5 for an extended period before they can wait to reach a 3 before they eat. Support Rita as she recognizes her fear of hunger while eating.

Case Study (Figure 4-F)

Tilly does not tolerate hunger and to make sure she does not get below a 5, she eats frequently, and to a fullness level of 9 or 10. Tilly tends to avoid discomfort in her life, and since being needy is uncomfortable, she spends much time helping others and avoiding her own needs. Ironically, she usually tends to be good at dieting because she gets caught up in the "high" of the diet, feeling better physically because she is not eating to 9 or 10. Eventually, she becomes unable to ignore her hunger and her needs, finding both intolerable. She falls off the diet, and continues to find hunger intolerable. Tilly is prone to getting "stuck" in therapy by not taking action and focusing session time on others' needs. She is frightened of discussing her own needs, even when her life is not working well.

Treatment strategy: In a session, have Tilly wait to reach level 4 on the scale before eating and process this experience. Model a nonjudgmental style of sharing. Encourage Tilly to share her fears of being hungry and discuss what her body feels like at a 4. When she can wait until level 4 to eat most of the time, bring the fullness number down one level (e.g. from 10 to 9). Have Tilly work toward eating between levels 3 and 7 or 8. She may benefit from understanding physiologically that it is normal and healthy to allow her body to get hungry. Tilly may be hesitant and afraid to change and will benefit from close support and encouragement.

Case Study (Figure 4-G)

Jess discovers that his level of fullness continues to increase even after he finishes eating or he is unable to stop eating before feeling uncomfortably full. Jess may be easily distracted during a meal leaving him less attentive to physical cues of satisfaction or fullness building towards the end of the meal.

Treatment strategy: Have Jess record his level of fullness halfway through the meal, upon completion of the meal, and then again 10-15 minutes later. If the fullness level increases, he will benefit from techniques designed to slow down the eating process. Encourage him to eat to a 5 or 6 and take a "wait and see" attitude. This could be done in a session together (21).

Identify Emotional "Hunger" Using the Hunger Scale

Use the Hunger Scale to help identify "emotional hunger." After exploring the client's perception of physical and emotional hunger, ask the client to chart the emotional hunger directly beneath the physical hunger, possibly with a different marking in the squares as in Connie's journal below. This helps to separate emotions from physical hunger. (Be sure to help clients identify the impact stress, illness, menstrual cycle, physical activity, and medications have on their physical cues.)

Case Study (Figure 4-H)

Coleen is aware of her emotions as shown by the squares marked (/ / / /). She does not feel entitled to eat if she has feelings, and so she denies her hunger, meaning she denies her needs. It may be too overwhelming for Coleen to feel emotional needs and physical needs at the same time.

Figure 4-F   TILLY'S FOOD JOURNAL

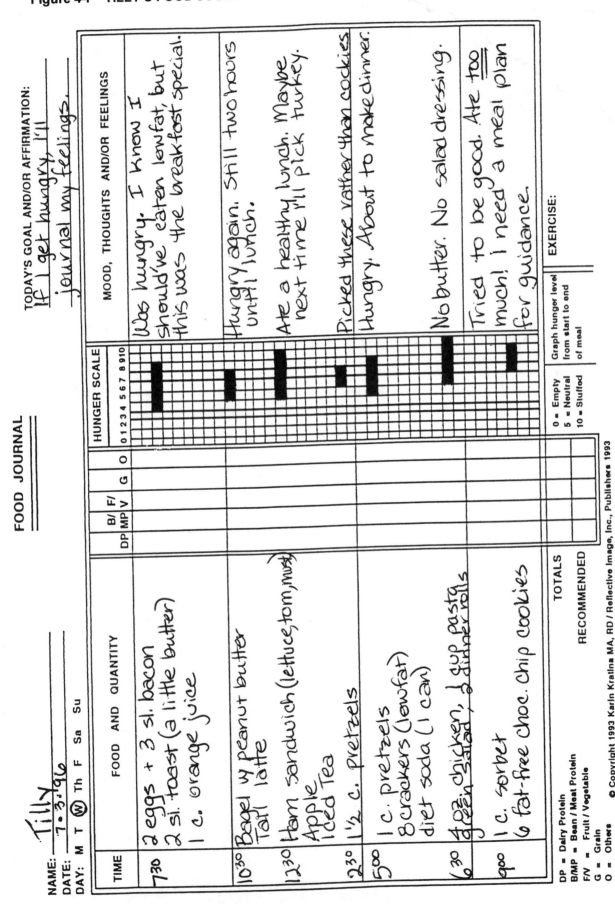

Figure 4-G   JESS' FOOD JOURNAL

FOOD JOURNAL

NAME: Jess

DATE: 9.9.96

DAY: (M) T W Th F Sa Su

TODAY'S GOAL AND/OR AFFIRMATION: Notice how much food I need to be satisfied/full.

TIME	FOOD AND QUANTITY	DP	B/ MP	F/ V	G	O	HUNGER SCALE 0 1 2 3 4 5 6 7 8 9 10	MOOD, THOUGHTS AND/OR FEELINGS
6:30	Coffee (2 large cups) Breakfast Burrito (Grande)							Ate in car on way to work. Very fast. But it was good. Got really full.
1:30	Roastbeef sandwich Iced tea (large) Small cup of potato salad							In my car again. Making cold calls to prospective clients. Ugh! Should have gotten 6" sandwich not 12" felt fine halfway thru
8:30	Chips and salsa Fish tacos Lite beer (ordered a second beer)							Felt great at a (7). Second beer and more chips sent me to a (10).
11:45	Ø							Tired. Comfortable finally. I like going to bed feeling at a (5).
	TOTALS						Graph hunger level from start to end of meal	EXERCISE: Fun!! Basketball (1½ hrs)
	RECOMMENDED						0 = Empty 5 = Neutral 10 = Stuffed	

DP = Dairy Protein
B/MP = Bean / Meat Protein
F/V = Fruit / Vegetable
G = Grain
O = Others

Figure 4-H   COLEEN'S FOOD JOURNAL

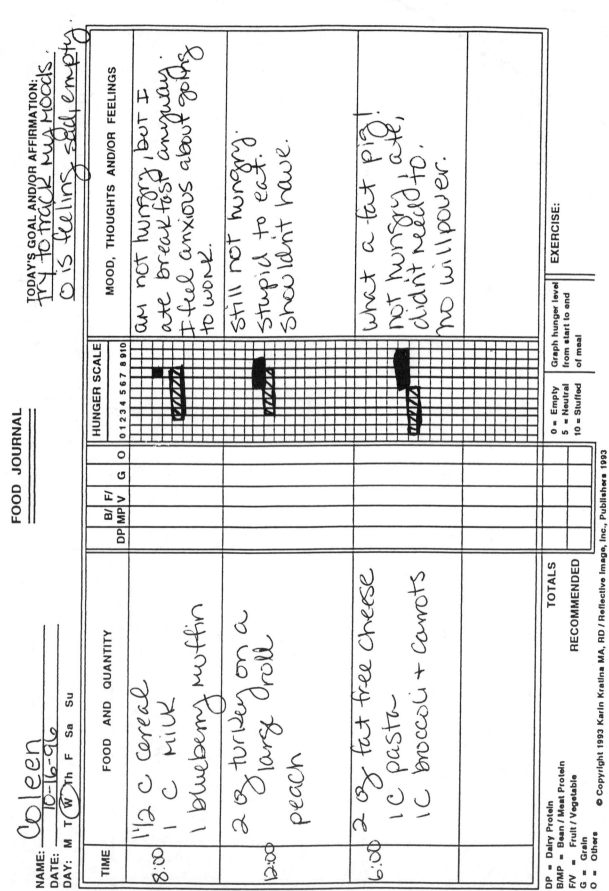

Or, she may believe having needs implies some kind of weakness or lack of self-sufficiency. She turns feelings of resentment and frustration about having needs inward and engages in negative self-talk.

Treatment Strategy: Guide Coleen in exploring fullness from a physical standpoint and compare these levels to 5,4,3, etc. Given the amount of food she ate the day of the record, it does not make sense she would feel that full. In addition, you can affirm that feelings are normal and so is hunger. This is foundational in order for Coleen to eventually come to accept her needs.

Keep in mind changes usually occur slowly. Clients may be able to tolerate changing only one meal each week. Most clients take three to four weeks to begin feeling comfortable working with the concept of the Hunger Scale. The more the Hunger Scale is reinforced in sessions with your clients, the quicker they will incorporate it into their daily experiences.

SUMMARY

By shifting from the paradigm of selecting food based on external direction, clients are guided in exploring, their own physical experiences with food, including food's impact on their health in a nonjudgmental environment. Clients become more insightful and inquisitive. Through being more introspective they learn much more about themselves. Clients become able to identify their own problematic eating behaviors, express how they feel about them, and tap into a genuine desire for information and solutions. Rather than acting as authority figures and directors, you guide. Carefully and attentively, you assess the clients' preferred eating style and intake for nutritional adequacy, health risk reduction, and total health promotion.

Each client has his or her own history, health status, goals, and preferences. You explore with them, empowering them to ask for themselves, "Is this food choice a health enhancing one for me physically, spiritually (23), emotionally, mentally and socially?"

Note: Although a thorough discussion of hunger and satiety research is beyond the scope of this manual, health care providers working in the nondiet paradigm may find their skills and understanding greatly enhanced by staying current. It is the authors' hope that interest in the nondiet paradigm will prompt even further research in this complex area.

SELECTED RESOURCES

Breaking the Diet Habit. Janet Polivy, Peter Herman. New York, NY: Basic Books; 1983.
Written by well-known researchers in the area of food restriction, this books gives practical guidelines on how to develop a normal eating style while ending the dieting cycle.

Intuitive Eating, A Recovery Book for the Chronic Dieter. Evelyn Tribole, Elyse Resch. New York, NY: St. Martin's Press; 1995.
A refreshing and enjoyable book aimed at helping individuals discover and be guided by internal cues of hunger, fullness and satiety. The authors explain how to make peace with food by getting off the dieting cycle, and instead trusting the body's own intuition in making food choices.

Taste and The Feeding Experience. Disordered eating and assessment tools. Karin Kratina. Plantation, FL: Reflective Image, Inc.; 1993. (954) 370-0725
Camera-ready tools and handouts for use with clients with disordered eating.

Women and Hunger: The Non-Diet Approach to Reaching and Maintaining Your Natural Weight.
Karin Kratina, Iris Nystrom. Plantation, FL: Reflective Image, Inc.; 1993. (954) 370-0725
These two audio tapes focus on learning to eat when hungry and stop when satisfied. The listener is encouraged to end dieting and is given techniques to develop an internally-regulated eating style. The tapes provide relaxation methods and prompt listeners in getting in touch with hunger and satiety.

REFERENCES

1. Stacey M. *Consumed: Why Americans Love, Hate, and Fear Food.* New York, NY: Touchstone; 1994.

2. Funk P. *Standard Dictionary.* New York, NY: HarperCollins; 1993.

3. King NL, Kratina K, In the trenches: Dealing with the "fat-free backlash." *SCAN PULSE.* 1995; 14: 8-10.

4. Mock AD, MSW, LCSW. Personal communication. Child and family psychotherapist, Montrose, CA, June 21, 1996.

5. Kilpatrick, MA, MSW, BCD. Personal communication. Marriage and family psychotherapist, trauma consultant, La Canada Flintridge, CA, June 19, 1996.

6. Allred JB. Too much of a good thing: An overemphasis on eating low-fat foods may be contributing to the alarming increase in overweight among US adults. *J Am Diet Assoc.* 1995; 95: 417-418.

7. Capaldi ED, Powley TL editors. *Taste, Experience, and Feeding.* Washington, DC: APA; 1990.

8. Drewnowski A. Fats and food acceptance: sensory, hedonic and attitudinal aspects. In: Solms J, Booth DA, Pangborn RM, Raunhardt O, eds. *Food Acceptance and Nutrition.* New York, NY: Academic Press; 1988: 189-204.

9. Rolls BJ, Kim-Harris S, Fischman MW, Foltin RW, MoranTH, Stoner SA. Satiety after preloads with different amounts of fat and carbohydrate: Implications for obesity. *Am J of Clin Nutr.* 1994; 60:476-487.

10. Blundell JE, Lawton CL, Hill AJ. Mechanisms of appetite control and their abnormalities in obese patients. *Horm-Res.* 1993; 39S: 72-76.

11. Rolls BJ, Dimeo KA, Shide DJ. Age-related impairments in the regulation of food intake. *Am J Clin Nutr.* 1995; 62: 923-931.

12. Polivy J. Psychological consequences of food restriction. *J Am Diet Assoc.* 1996; 96:589-592.

13. America's weight problem: What are we doing about it? *Calorie Control Commentary.* 1996; 18:1-2.

14. Mellin LM, Scully S, Irwin CE. Disordered eating characteristics in preadolescent girls. Paper presented at the *American Dietetic Association Annual Meeting and Exhibition,* Las Vegas, NV 1986.

15. Johnson CL, Tobiu DL, Lipkin J. Epidemiologic changes in bulimic behavior among female adolescents over a five-year period. *Intnatl J of Eating Disord.* 1989; 8: 647-655.

16. Bloom C, Gitter A, Gutwill S, Kogel L, Zaphiropoulos L. *Eating Problems: A Feminist Psychoanalytic Treatment Model.* New York, NY: Basic Books; 1994.

17. Kratina K. The Food/Feelings Journal in: *Disordered Eating Assessment and Treatment Tools.* Plantation, FL: Reflective Image, Inc.; 1993.

18. Keys A, Brozek J, Henschel A, Mickelson O', Taylor HL. *The Biology of Human Starvation. 2 vols.* Minneapolis: University of Minnesota Press; 1950.

19. Rolls BJ, Carbohydrates, fats, and satiety, *Am J Clin Nutr.* 1995; 61S: 960S-967S.

20. Kerr D, Sherwin RS, Paralkis F, et al. Effect of caffeine on the recognition and responses to hypoglycemia in humans. *Ann Intern. Med.* 1993; 119: 799-804.

21. King NL, DeMars P, Kratina K. HungerWork: Returning to physically-connected eating. *SCAN PULSE.* 1996; 15: 12-14.

22. Martini MC, Lampe JW, Slavin JL, Kurzer MS. Effect of the menstrual cycle on energy and nutrient intake. *Am J Clin Nutr.* 1994; 60:895-899.

23. Goldman C. The Power of Prayer in Medicine. *Diab Self-Management.* 1995; Sept/Oct: 24-27.

Moving Away From Diets
A Personal Perspective

My name is Joanna M. I'm 53 years old, a psychotherapist and college instructor, now living in Tacoma, Washington. I have been working with Nancy King, MS, RD, CDE, nutrition therapist, for the last two years.

What personal experiences led you to move to a nondieting paradigm?

I weighed 11 lbs., 13 oz. at birth. Both my parents and 3 of my 4 siblings are considerably overweight. I remember being called "fatty" from the time I began school and began my first diet shortly thereafter. I have spent a lifetime dieting and have done everything from pills, fasting (literally), fasting with a supplement in a supervised program through UCLA, the Stillman Diet, the Atkins Diet, a diet in which I drank an ounce of safflower oil before every meal, to finally just giving up and saying, "what the heck." I have lost thousands of pounds in my lifetime, including 150 pounds two different times and gained it all back and more. I came to realize that diets simply do not work. As a result of the fasting supplement program, I developed gall bladder disease and had to have my gall bladder removed. I almost died during this process due to complications from pancreatitis. I forgot to mention O.A., TOPS, Weight Watchers (at least 6 times), etc.

I have also fallen prey to the "plastic surgery" trap. I had sagging skin removed from both upper arms and forearms and liposuction done on them, in a total of 5 different surgeries. I have major scaring on one arm that looks worse than a burn scar and will probably never go away. I also had a roll of skin (from gaining and losing weight so many times) removed from my abdomen. Liposuction was used as well. Again, there were complications from the surgery and I had to have a second major surgery three months later to have a penrose drain removed which had gotten sucked up into my abdomen. Again the doctor did liposuction and my abdomen is very asymmetrical and will never look normal. My naval is also only about 2 inches from my pubic area now.

During all of these procedures, I was saying all the right words. I am not sorry to be rid of the roll of skin from my abdomen, as it was a constant source of discomfort. However, the reality is that I was desperate--I would do anything to be "normal". Of course, I am still very obese and not "normal".

In the past, I have been on extensive exercise programs from time to time. For over a year, I played singles tennis on a daily basis and then swam a mile 4 times a week. Then I would go home and ride my bicycle for 1/2 hour. All the time, I was stopping to make sure that my heartbeat was at the appropriate target rate. Another time I went to the gym on a daily basis and worked out for 1 1/2 hours a day.

In a video on nondieting called "Body Trust: Undieting Your Weigh to Health and Happiness," a woman made the comment that she had dieted her way to 300 pounds. I, too, had dieted my way to 300 pounds. Now, my weight has settled in about 25 pounds less than that and for the time being that is okay.

The BBTs (bad body thoughts) are such an overwhelming part of obesity, that simply eating oneself silly doesn't work either. It is just the opposite end of the dieting spectrum. In my opinion, there must be some kind of balance between noticing what's going on in your body, noticing what you are eating, noticing what kind of movement your body wants and needs, and just "legalizing" and EATING everything in sight. I really like the term I have heard instead of legalizing--"neutralizing" food--simply not making it good or bad.

What experiences have you had with health care professionals?

I have been humiliated by health care professionals most of my life. I have experienced everything from a doctor (who was considerably overweight himself) poking me in the stomach and telling me I needed to lose weight, to a doctor performing a procedure on my leg telling me that I was gross, to having an x-ray technician telling me that I was "way too big to get in the picture."

I shared an article on obese people working with doctors in a partnership regarding their own healthcare, by Art Patterson (Speaking Patiently, pages 13-14), with a friend who was a physician and he was quite moved by it and wanted to know if he had ever done any of those things to me. I told him, "no." But, it gave us an opportunity to dialogue about the subject. He noted that for most of us who are obese, we filter everything through a filter that says we need to lose weight. So, when he says, increase your exercise, the obese person is hearing, and he is in effect saying, "lose weight." When he says to a diabetic, "cut down on your sugar" he is again saying, "lose weight." My physician friend came up with about 15 different ways he has said "lose weight" without ever saying, lose weight. He made multiple copies of the article and made it required reading for all of his staff and said he was going to share it with as many of his colleagues as he could.

How do you define whether or not you have been successful with a nondiet approach?
I have stopped dieting and believe I have been successful. This is not to say that I don't still want desperately to lose weight. However, it does not control my life. Instead, I am more in tune with my body. Now, much of the time, I eat things because I want to, and am not controlled by them. For example, I have been known to sit down and eat 2 large pizzas at one setting. Now I am more apt to eat 2 pieces of pizza, know that it will still be there tomorrow, and I can have more then.

I was never aware of feeling full, because I was not totally in touch with my body. Through therapy and work with my nutrition therapist, I have begun to feel my body and know more what it wants. I now am able to know when I am full. I don't believe there are foods that I can't have. However, I am more apt to have a few bites of cheesecake, instead of a whole cheesecake or even a whole piece of cheesecake. I am more aware of wanting to put healthy foods into my body. I still struggle with "fast food." Sometimes when I look at what I have eaten, it is not large quantities, but rather it is simply fast food as opposed to food I have cooked myself.

I have been very resistant to exercise. Again, it represented all of the same things which were represented by dieting. Now, I move my body in ways which are pleasant for me and yet still give me exercise. I love to dance--and have taken as many as four dance classes a week, as well as going dancing on the weekend. I also love to play tennis and swim. These are things which do not feel like "exercise" to me. Rather they are things I like to do.

I must be honest and tell you that I go "in and out" of these things. However, I feel that I eat on this level far more often than not. One way that I believe I can determine I have been successful with this "nondiet" approach is that my weight has stabilized. I have remained within about 5 pounds of the same weight for approximately 6 months now. When I do decide to cut down on my food intake, I don't attempt to "diet" myself into starvation. Rather I have been losing approximately 1/2 to 1 pound a week.

Has using a nondiet approach changed your life? In what ways?
I'm not sure whether using the nondiet approach or working with the nutrition therapist has been what has changed my life. Actually, the two are inseparable, I guess. The therapist's nonjudgmental acceptance has been invaluable. As a result, I am far more accepting of myself. While there are times I still struggle with depression and feeling badly about myself, my self-esteem has risen incredibly. I am far more willing and able to be "out there" with people and let my own self shine through.

I believe so strongly in this approach, that as a therapist, I am in the process of putting together a group on self-acceptance and self-esteem for obese persons. Obviously, many of the things I have learned in this personal journey will be the basis for attempting to help participants in this group. I truly believe that this is a lifestyle change for me. I can't imagine ever starving myself to lose weight again. I have now become far more aware when I am eating out of deprivation and try to stay in touch with my body's needs.

5

HUNGER WORK:
Heal Disconnected Eating

> *Clients may say, "Who am I? Who will I be if I do not diet? Can I do this radical, almost anti-female act of eating what I want? Can I really have, and am I really entitled to this bountifulness? Do I really deserve this kind of self-acceptance? I don't trust my insides. I know what food is nutritious, but I can't be trusted to eat it (1)."*

IDENTIFY AND DECODE EATING EXPERIENCES

Eating Styles

The second facet of HungerWork is healing disconnected eating, which begins with a discussion of the three major types of eating. Included are descriptions of each eating style and treatment strategies and techniques to help clients reconnect to internal cues, particularly those engaged in deprivation-driven eating and emotional or compulsive eating. Decoding eating experiences includes exploring beyond the eating behavior to understand the function of the behavior. Chapter 8 "Concepts in Action" addresses decoding extensively.

#1 Physically-connected eating (natural eating) This person eats most of the time in response to internal cues of hunger and fullness. Physically-connected eaters may present with a desire to eat more healthfully, improve self-management of a nutrition-sensitive disease, or tailor their eating style to better support physical activity. These clients are most receptive to utilizing nutrition information delivered in a nonjudgmental, explorative environment.

#2 Deprivation-driven eating This person's drive to eat stems from having been restricted or limited from the food he or she wants or needs. Deprivation can manifest itself physically from not providing necessary foods for health and well-being. It can also manifest psychologically by not having freedom to eat the way one wants to, or being criticized or judged for eating the way one wants to. In short, the deprivation-driven eater has been deprived of satisfaction from food.

#3 Emotional/compulsive eating This person's drive originates in having thoughts and feelings that he or she cannot identify, accept, express, care for, tolerate, or resolve. The individual feels compelled to seek something outside of him/herself to distract, cover up, or push down feelings; anything to change the way he or she feels inside. Unfortunately, the substance or behavior chosen does not keep the feelings or thoughts away permanently, nor does it resolve the original distress or the present conflict. But, because the food is temporarily soothing and no alternative is seen, the behavior continues.

Differentiating between these three main types of eating will help you identify and assess clients' needs. In turn, you will be able to select appropriate treatment strategies and techniques to help them reconnect to their internal cues. It also helps your clients understand the origin and evolution of their eating problems.

Note that deprivation-driven eating and emotional or compulsive eating both originate from the pain of unrecognized and unmet needs. They exacerbate each other, but do not always accompany each other in disconnected eating. For example, a client may eat physically-connected for breakfast, lunch, and dinner (pattern #1), but eat for emotional reasons (pattern #3) late at night. Another may settle for fat free potato chips, eventually bingeing on the regular kind (pattern #2). Or, a client may restrict food all day, drinking coffee, eating a small salad at lunch (#2), then by dinner time be driven to eat due to hunger (#1) and subsequently binge from the stress of their workday (#2, #3). Two vital tools in determining the type(s) of eating they are engaged in are:

1. Inquiring specifically about clients' encounters and experiences with food and their bodies.
2. Utilizing food journals for more information about physical cues, food choices, and feelings.

#1 PHYSICALLY-CONNECTED EATING

Characteristics of physically-connected eating:
- eating for vitality, health, and enjoyment;
- eating in response to internal cues, nonrestrained;
- tempering choices with scientific nutrition facts.

Topics to enhance physically-connected eating:
- quality of nutrition information and affirmation;
- nutrition's role in reducing health risks;
- physical activity and health (i.e. physical health, emotional, mental, spiritual, and social);
- meal mix and expected outcome;
- nutrition, physical activity and nutrition-sensitive diseases;
- promote size acceptance, pleasurable eating, and joyful movement.

#2 DEPRIVATION-DRIVEN EATING

Characteristics of deprivation-driven eating:
- occurs when individual has not had free access to desired foods (or guilt-free access);
- results naturally from dieting and weight cycling;
- can escalate when following a special medical diet nutrition regimen;
- often borne of, and perpetuated by, labeling food as "good" and "bad."

Effective approaches for healing deprivation-driven eating:
- lift restrictions and moralization off of food;
- know where the next meal, or snack is coming from;
- teach and guide client to identify internal cues;
- shift from "responsible" eating to responsive eating;
- explore meal mix and expected outcome;
- promote size acceptance, pleasurable eating, and joyful movement.

Note: Deprivation driven eating *may* worsen with programs that place limits directly on the food or frequency of eating, such as: twelve-step programs *with eating plans*, medical diets, any nutrition regimen, diet, gram or calorie counting approaches.

Treatment Strategies and Techniques for Deprivation-Driven Eating
Deprivation-driven eaters often present desperately wanting a food plan or diet. They insist that this time they can adhere to it, in spite of their personal history and scientific research indicating otherwise. As you listen to the clients' convincing stories about how it will be different this time, you may feel inclined to support them in following a "reasonable, healthy diet"...nothing drastic. However, this is reinforcing the same belief system that worsens the sense of deprivation. Any approach which restricts the individual from the foods they desire will perpetuate the side effects of dieting: food preoccupation, overeating or bingeing, and increased emotional responsiveness (2,3). Following are strategies and techniques you can use to provide guidance and structure without restriction or chaos.

Provide Structure for Deprivation-Driven Eating. When moving away from diets, many clients feel unstable and insecure without the structure of a diet. You can assess degree and type of structure needed and provide it without returning to the diet paradigm. Nondiet work naturally varies in goal-orientation depending on clients' needs. Generally speaking, clients engaged in deprivation- driven eating benefit from less structure and more permission and encouragement to venture outside of their restrictive eating styles.

There are many nondiet approaches that heal deprivation-driven eating. Fundamentally, however, they all support and empower the client to make their own food choices in a nonmoralized context. Notice in the examples below working with the deprivation-driven eater, the focus is on providing an opportunity to begin trusting their internal cues and taking the authority to be the decision-maker.

A one-week goal for the client engaged in deprivation-driven eating could be: "I will monitor my body's cues and respond to physical hunger, fullness, and satiety. I will eat enough lunch to begin feeling some fullness pressure in my stomach." Another option could be: "I will decide what I really want to eat at two different meals this week. I will seek out that food and give myself permission to have it."

Make Food Available At All Times. Remind your clients that there is virtually an endless supply of food in this society. Most often, within a short period of time, foods of their choosing can be in their hands. When clients feel hungry, the natural, healthful, healing response is to eat. Not eating when hungry can be as profoundly disconnecting and detrimental as eating when one is not hungry.

One of the most profound ways to empower clients to feed themselves when they want, what they want, and the amount they want is a food bag. Having continual access to food can promote healing from deprivation-driven eating by providing a way for clients to feed themselves whenever their bodies indicate it is time to do so. Being able to provide food for oneself when the need arises allows for self-regulation, creates self-sufficiency, and fosters self-trust, and in turn reconnection.

❖ **Filling the Food Bag**
Contents of the bag can include previously restricted foods, foods for fuel, foods to handle hypoglycemic episodes (especially clients with diabetes), and favorite foods. The bag's contents and replenishment are the clients' responsibility. It may also be meaningful for clients to receive a gift of food (possibly from the health care provider) to put in the bag. Allowing ample time in a session for brainstorming can open up new possibilities as clients make a shopping list of foods for their bag.

❖ **Fears of Carrying "Too Much" in the Food Bag**
When starting out, some clients may fear carrying "too much food" in their food bag. Exploring what "too much" means can reveal clients' perceived tendency to binge or overeat. Recognize they are trying to protect themselves from "overeating" or losing control, a behavior they believe and experience as self-destructive. (The nondiet approach views this compensatory behavior as an attempt to return to normal eating.) Overtime, as a result of

lifting restrictive eating, this tendency will diminish. "Too much" could also mean any of the following:

- They may not trust their ability to assess their food needs.
- They may not trust their bodies' cues to stop eating.
- They may have distorted ideas of how much food their bodies need to be healthy.
- They may be looking entirely to the health care provider to decide the contents of the food bag.*

*Caution: This may be a variation of asking for another externally-directed food plan. Supporting clients in choosing the foods for their bags is helpful. However, in order for them to break out of the diet mentality, you must refrain from making the food choices for them.

Consider the Client's Needs and Capabilities. Some clients may not be able to think of more than two or three foods to carry. This could be a reflection of the restrictive food choices they have been operating within. It is important to meet clients where they are. If carrying only two or three items is their limit, start with that. With continual reassurance that feeding oneself is a right and a necessity, clients are eventually able to carry ample pleasurable provisions in the food bag. Often a food bag is the first experience clients have in providing sustenance for themselves. They may prefer to work on the food bag concept first to gain trust and confidence, then apply this same type of permission-giving and provision to approaching meals. *(Overcoming Overeating* by Carol Munter and Jane Hirschmann has an in-depth discussion of the food bag concept [4].)

#3 EMOTIONAL, COMPULSIVE EATING

Characteristics of emotional, compulsive eating:
- seeking something outside self to change inside self;
- eating is used to comfort, numb, express, stuff, distract;
- food is used as a companion;
- eating behavior has served as a survival tool, a coping skill;
- emotional eating behavior is exacerbated by deprivation.

Effective approaches for healing emotional, compulsive eating:
- track hunger or fullness;
- identify feeling states that prompt eating;
- support client in experiencing and expressing his or her feelings;
- include adjunct psychotherapy to process issues and feelings;
- contract to abstain from food behavior that client uses to hide feelings;
- consider support for abstinence from twelve-step or Behavior Change Contract (pg.74);
- promote size acceptance, pleasurable eating, and joyful movement.

Note: Emotional, compulsive eating covers up deeper feelings. In the process of dealing with food, weight, and body issues, clients discover emotions and behaviors that may need to be processed with a mental health professional. Be prepared to refer clients to psychotherapists (with nondiet philosophy) for adjunctive therapy.

Treatment Strategies and Techniques for Emotional, Compulsive Eating
While deprivation-driven eaters benefit, in general, from less structure around the food, the emotional,

compulsive eater benefits, in general, from *more* structure around food behaviors, particularly intense emotional eating times. This facilitates greater learning about what drives the emotional eating.

Provide Structure to Learn About Emotionally Prompted Eating

For the client engaged in compulsive, emotional eating, a one week goal could be:

(Client with diabetes and emotional eating) "I will self-monitor blood glucose levels and sense of well-being throughout the afternoon into dinner time, because I tend to binge eat from 1:00-5:00 p.m." Another option could be: "On my way home from work I will take an inventory of my feelings and pick two that I need to express to my husband before I walk into the kitchen to prepare dinner."

Once a client can accept structure around emotional eating episodes, two important changes begin to take shape:

1. They begin to experience their feelings more directly as the "covering" eating behavior is lifted.
2. They begin to experience the food as less chaotic and out of control, providing some relief from their distress (physical and emotional) over the eating.

Note: Professional supervision from a mentoring dietitian or psychotherapist can be extremely helpful in assessing and tailoring structure that suits clients' needs.

Recognize That Their Feelings Are Out of Control, Not the Food

Exploring clients' emotional eating reveals that it is not the food that is not out of control, but feelings that feel out of control. However, they perceive the food is the problem because it is used to cover, control, calm, or soothe their feelings. When emotional, compulsive eaters feel extremely chaotic, panicked, or out of control, and are eating to cover these feelings, they desire extreme structure to regain control. Many emotional, compulsive eaters opt to diet to satisfy this need for structure.

Following a diet, by design, does not present many extraneous eating opportunities to cover up feelings with food. The feelings that are now "uncovered" may be so painful that individuals feel compelled to eat to distract themselves from these feelings. They may also want to "numb out" by consuming great quantities of carbohydrates (5). Actually, in very real terms they are abandoning themselves because of the intensity of their own feelings. This is a deeply painful form of rejection.

#2 DEPRIVATION-DRIVEN EATING COMBINED with #3 EMOTIONAL, COMPULSIVE EATING

Characteristics of deprivation-driven eating combined with emotional, compulsive eating:
- very common combination of eating styles;
- eating serves to cope with emotions;
- history of restrained eating;
- feels, initially, like nonrestrained eating style exacerbates the compulsive eating;
- feels chaotic and out of control;
- desires structure to come from outside of themselves;
- lacks trust in own judgment to self-manage food.

Effective approaches for healing deprivation-driven and emotional, compulsive eating:
- maintain nonrestrained eating atmosphere as much as possible;
- look for eating behavior that is prompted by emotions that need new boundaries;
- recognize food is not out of control, resist structuring the food;
- track hunger/fullness on Hunger Scale, track emotional hunger just below physical (see example of Coleen on page 62);
- acknowledge feelings or lack of connection with self, use psychotherapy for support;
- promote size acceptance, pleasurable eating, and joyful movement.

Treatment Strategies and Techniques for Deprivation-Driven Eating Combined with Emotional, Compulsive Eating

The following case study illustrates these two eating styles in combination. Within the study the following treatment strategies and techniques have been highlighted so you can easily identify them:
- Recommend adjunct psychotherapy.
- Support responding to internal cues.
- Promote nonrestrained eating.
- Differentiate between two styles of disconnected eating.
- Neutralize the food.
- Inquire about physical experience.
- Identify emotional eating behavior.
- Utilize a behavior change contract.
- Place structure around emotional eating behavior.
- Provide nonjudgmental support.
- Incorporate the food/feelings journal.

Note: The terms "emotional eating" and "compulsive eating" are used interchangeably. Binge eating can be triggered by deprivation or emotions.

Case Study: Andrea

Andrea is 31 years old, married, and has two young children. She worked weekly with a dietitian in a nondiet approach for six months of this past year. Her goal has been to eliminate diet cycling and binge eating. At the six month mark, the **dietitian recommended a psychotherapist for Andrea and her husband** to deal with relationship issues that came up in nutrition counseling, which are outside the scope of a dietitian's practice. Soon after she started marriage counseling, Andrea, her therapist, and her dietitian agreed that she needed to devote more time to her marriage issues and put the nutrition work "on hold" to prevent therapy overload.

Andrea had learned to focus on **eating from internal cues in a nonrestrained fashion**. As a result, her **deprivation-driven eating** was practically nonexistent. However, due to the difficult feelings that came up in marriage counseling, she experienced a significant increase in **emotional eating**. She felt panicked and frightened since she had **neutralized** all food and had no external rules to govern her eating. This lack of external authority made her feel like she had free reign to compulsively eat.

Andrea knew therapy had been hard and she had some understanding as to why her feelings trigger compulsive eating. However, because of her chaotic eating, she desired structure around the food. Although Andrea had always turned to dieting when she started eating emotionally, she now saw dieting as the cause of deprivation-driven eating and it was no longer an option. Nonetheless, she was at a loss and feared there was no other solution to calm the chaotic eating.

Now after a six month hiatus, and at the suggestion of her therapist, Andrea returns to her dietitian for help. Restricting Andrea's access to the foods she wants, would not only trigger deprivation-driven eating, but would negatively impact the therapeutic relationship. The dietitian would become to Andrea: 1) the one she is supposed to please by sticking to the diet, but will disappoint when she goes off it, or 2) the one she is resentful of and rebels against.

The dietitian consults with the therapist (written permission secured from Andrea to do so) and learns Andrea has a greater sense of herself, is more in touch with her feelings, and has strengthened her ability to feel her feelings and express them.

Although Andrea knows she is not food deprived and is not engaged in negative self-talk, **she feels bad physically from the recent compulsive eating episodes.** Her pattern has been to **eat chocolate or cookies in the late afternoon to numb herself before her husband comes home from work.** In light of how poorly she feels physically and emotionally, Andrea decides she is motivated to explore whether or not she can get through the late afternoon without bingeing.

Because Andrea has become so attuned to her physical cues, she is less tolerant of the groggy, exhausted way she feels after the compulsive eating episodes. She recognizes this numbing is about disconnecting from her feelings, abandoning her feelings, and therefore, abandoning herself. Furthermore, because Andrea has been in psychotherapy working on healthy ways to deal with feelings, she is motivated and equipped to confront the issues, thoughts, and feelings that the afternoon compulsive eating behavior is hiding.

Andrea and her dietitian agree to draw up a contract (6), Figure 5-A, identifying the behavior she wishes to abstain from. The purpose is to learn more about herself while breaking the afternoon compulsive eating cycle. **Andrea suggests avoiding the eating behavior that she uses to disconnect from her feelings in the afternoon.**

Note: The dietitian and therapist both encourage Andrea to explore and discover her feelings, without criticism or judgment. If Andrea breaks the contract she knows **both health care providers will remain nonjudgmental and supportive**.

At her next session with the dietitian Andrea reports, "So far it is going well. I feel good. Over the last two days I have experienced the freedom and confidence that comes from trusting myself again. I am able to have what I want to eat throughout the day because I am able to keep my word in the afternoon, abstaining from "checking out" in order to be with my feelings. And I learned the most incredible thing about myself...when the painful feelings come, they last all of 10 seconds. Sometimes they come often, kind of like in waves, but I can either sit through them, journal them, talk into my recorder, or share them with a friend."

For the past six weeks, Andrea has initiated reviewing and renewing her behavior change contract with the dietitian This is a sign she may be ready to self-monitor her structure in the afternoon. She says, "Lately when I think of disconnecting from my feelings in the afternoon, I can picture going through the feelings, staying with myself, and guiding myself out of them with support from those close to me. The previous behavior felt so bad physically. I felt so sad and abandoned emotionally. Why do that to myself? It feels so freeing that I no longer have to."

Andrea, by her own suggestion, is now using a food/feelings journal to express the feelings that had been covered by the emotional eating. She takes this journal to therapy to help knit together the work she is doing with the therapist and the dietitian.

Andrea's Results

Three important things happened for Andrea on that first afternoon she was willing to abstain from compulsive eating:

1. She discovered some of her true feelings hidden by food. Some feelings did not last as long as she thought they would.
2. She was able to stay with and not abandon herself. Therefore she was able to begin rebuilding trust in herself and provide needed structure.
3. She forged ahead in therapy to disconnect the feelings from her eating behavior so she can express and deal with them.

Figure 5-A ANDREA'S BEHAVIOR CHANGE CONTRACT

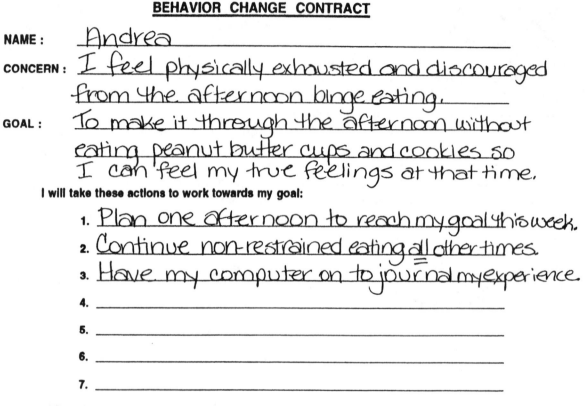

BEHAVIOR CHANGE CONTRACT

NAME : Andrea

CONCERN : I feel physically exhausted and discouraged from the afternoon binge eating.

GOAL : To make it through the afternoon without eating peanut butter cups and cookies so I can feel my true feelings at that time.

I will take these actions to work towards my goal:

1. Plan one afternoon to reach my goal this week.
2. Continue non-restrained eating all other times.
3. Have my computer on to journal my experience.
4. _____
5. _____
6. _____
7. _____

Check box when above actions accomplished:

	Day 1	Day 2	Day 3	Day 4	Day 5	Day 6	Day 7
1							
2							
3							
4							
5							
6							
7							

I have established a goal and constructive actions to reach my goal. I am committed to follow through with this plan for the next seven days.

Andrea W.   Dietitian
Signature   Co-signed
Date: 6-12-96

In this treatment approach, the focus is not on what Andrea is eating, but rather on the issues that arise when she adheres to the contract and abstaining from the specific compulsive behavior.

CREATIVE IDEAS FOR FURTHER CLIENT SUPPORT

Additional support may be helpful when clients are at the critical "crossroads" of feeling driven to engage in the compulsive behavior versus getting through the feeling without it. When you cannot be available for this additional support, clients can journal their feelings, record on a hand held recorder (bring it to next session), talk on your voice mail or answering machine (providing it is confidential), schedule a phone appointment, or increase frequency of sessions. Being alone with these feelings can be discouraging and overwhelming. Connecting with another individual to share feelings at this turning point can provide significant support.

PSYCHOTHERAPY TO BREAK THE CYCLE

Psychotherapy is vitally important so clients can learn about their feelings and how to care for them. If clients are involved in HungerWork but do not know how to deal with feelings, the following cycle may get entrenched:

1) they abstain from compulsive eating behavior,
2) their underlying feelings arise,
3) they feel afraid or ashamed for having feelings,
4) they do not know what to do with the feelings,
5) so they resort to compulsive eating to cover up feelings again.

Note: Some clients may find additional support in twelve-step and other self-help programs to cope without the compulsive behavior. **Not all self-help groups or therapy environments promote size acceptance and other aspects of the nondiet approach.** Some programs, such as Overeaters Anonymous, may have an overt or covert emphasis on weight loss as one of the primary measures of success. These programs have the potential to be compatible with psychotherapy and nutrition therapy. It is recommended the health care provider screen the group for compatible philosophies prior to clients joining.

SUMMARY

HungerWork creates the potential to provide clients with their first insight into how physical and emotional cues support or conversely interfere with their health goals. Learning how to respond to physical cues results in a greater sense of control over their body and food, and allows for self-trust to emerge. This reconnection decreases chaos around food and feelings. Clients can return to physically-connected eating and move away from deprivation-driven or emotional eating. As restraint is genuinely lifted from food, clients experience less intensity to binge from deprivation. By placing structure around emotional eating behaviors, clients experience and learn to care for feelings that used to be covered up by emotional eating. These techniques lead to breakthrough experiences that foster self-acceptance, self-trust, and reconnection.

SELECTED RESOURCES

Breaking Free From Compulsive Eating. Geneen Roth. Indianapolis: Bobbs-Merrill; 1984.

One of the first guide books for ending compulsive eating. Roth describes how compulsive eating takes root. She encourages the reader to see the eating behavior as an attempt to care for oneself, rather than self-recriminate. Roth provides seven guidelines an individual can consider each time they choose to eat. Using these guidelines allows an individual to experience food and eating in a noncompulsive fashion.

Consumed: Why Americans Love, Hate, and Fear Food. Michelle Stacey. New York, NY: Touchstone; 1994.

Through Stacey's humorous, quick-moving journalistic style, she explores and challenges America's belief systems and notions about food, especially "good and bad" food and what constitutes a healthy, pleasurable way to eat. A freeing approach is offered that eases fears and lifts obsessions about food, weight, health, and eating.

Eating Problems: A feminist psychoanalytic treatment model. C Bloom, A Gitter, S Gutwill, L Kogel, L Zaphiropoulos. New York, NY: BasicBooks; 1994.

A feminist perspective on the development and perpetuation of eating disorders, food fears, and body hatred. In-depth discussions from the therapist's viewpoint explore the functions of problematic food and body relationships, including treatment strategies and expected outcome. Self-care, self-nurture, and self-acceptance are fundamental to healing eating problems.

Making Peace With Food (**revised edition**). Susan Kano. New York, NY: Harper Row; 1989.

This is a workbook with exercises to reveal how attitudes and expressions become attached to food, eating, weight, body size, and exercise and ways to heal these painful connections. There is a section on the role family and friends can play in supporting the individual healing from problematic eating, exercise, and body image.

Overcoming Overeating. Jane Hirschmann , Carol Munter. New York, NY: Addison-Wesley; 1988.

An empowering approach to finding freedom from dieting, but particularly from deprivation-driven eating. Thoughtful attention is paid to diversity and size acceptance. Overcoming Overeating has gained international acceptance. Hirschmann and Munter offer retreats, seminars, newsletters and centers across the United States dedicated to promoting life free of diets and deprivation.

REFERENCES

1. Bloom C, Gitter A, Gutwill S, Kogel L, Zaphiropoulos L. *Eating Problems: A Feminist Psychoanalytic Treatment Model.* New York, NY: Basic Books; 1994.
2. Polivy J. Psychological consequences of food restriction. *J Am Diet Assoc.* 1996; 96:589-592.
3. White F. "The Dieting Cycle." Original illustration. Santa Barbara, CA: 1996.
4. Hirschmann JR, Munter CH. *Overcoming Overeating.* New York, NY: Ballantine Books; 1988.
5. Waterhouse D. *Why Women Need Chocolate.* New York, NY: Hyperion; 1995.
6. Kratina K. Behavior Change Contract in: *Disordered Eating Assessment and Treatment Tools.* Plantation, FL: Reflective Image, Inc.; 1993.

Moving Away From Diets
Personal/Professional Persceptives

Cheri E., Educator and Counselor, Illinois

Some people say that only frustrated professionals want this approach, that clients don't want it. UNTRUE! In my work with women of all sizes, but especially larger women who have been chronic dieters, I have found that they are frustrated and angry about having been given the same old tired solutions (dieting) over the years only to find themselves fatter than before they started to diet. The women I work with are hungry for a new way to relate to food, eating, and their health. When given permission to stop dieting and focus on healthy behaviors many of these women have regained not only their physical health but their self-esteem.

What personal/professional experiences led you to move to a nondieting paradigm?

PERSONAL: I was put on my first diet at age 5 and continued to diet until I was 38 years old. My weight ranged from 135-235 and I lost and gained at least 400 pounds in those three decades. I stopped dieting almost 10 years ago and my weight has stabilized in the higher weight range. All my vitals are normal. I have been a lap swimmer for 15 years. I tend to make "healthy" food choices because I feel more energy when I eat them, yet I do not deny myself anything I want to eat. The days of restricting and bingeing are over.

I have been liberated from the unhealthfulness of my dieting days, have maintained my weight, and am healthier than I have ever been. My self-esteem has also improved greatly in that I no longer feel shamed when a diet has failed me because I no longer "do food" in that way.

PROFESSIONAL: As an educator and counselor, I have been working with women of all sizes around this issue since 1982. As I became more enlightened around my own personal health related to food, dieting, body image, I began to share these ideas with my students and clients. I find that most women who come to my classes are afraid to stop dieting because they are afraid of food. I teach them this is a process and get them to focus on what they can do to increase their health and self-esteem--eat for health and pleasure, get their body moving, and get on with their lives. I have seen miracles happen with women who begin to listen to their bodies, trust their bodies and respond to their bodies in the gentle way of a nondieting approach.

What are the biggest challenges in working with a nondiet paradigm?
The biggest challenge was taking this idea seriously in my own life, and once I got that piece, it has been relatively easy to work with others. The problem with many professionals is that they themselves are restricting their eating and afraid of becoming fat. I believe that you can't teach this one without living it yourself. The professional who lives this is the strongest role model there is, and clients will respond with gusto!

What types of clients are best suited for a nondiet approach?
Because I have become a role model of health and fitness for larger women I have a tendency to attract other larger women who are really ready for this message. Lately I feel like I've been on "clean-up detail" from the survivors of Opti-Fast. I predict that in a couple of years nondieting professionals will once again be on "clean-up detail" from the survivors of Phen/fen and Redux. I think the nondiet approach is appropriate for any woman who wants to get healthy. I can't think of a population (even people with diabetes) who can't use this idea in their lives.

How do you work with other professionals/colleagues who may not be comfortable with a nondiet approach?

I have been so "out there" for so long about this that few people challenge me any more. I think the fact that I represent that which people think doesn't exist--health in a 200# body--puts me at an edge. I also think knowing the research that supports a "fat and fit/ healthy" mentality works well with the intellectual skeptics. I also throw in the "you grew up in this paradigm, too, and if you still hate your body, diet, etc., then you will have a hard time understanding and helping others who want to move on." A little guilt (did I say that?) never hurt. It gets people thinking about their own lives, attitudes, and how they contribute to the problem. It gets them at the emotional level, and for women especially, we have to deal this out emotionally as well as intellectually. (Of course, I am a therapist so I would want to mention the emotional components to this problem in other helpers.)

What words of wisdom do you have for those who are beginning to explore a nondiet paradigm?

READ, READ, READ all the research supporting a "health comes in all sizes" paradigm. Then think about how your personal life reflects your attitude about your own body, food issues, fat phobia, etc., and begin to work there. Talk to fat people and get to know them and listen to their stories and take them seriously. If a fat woman says she doesn't eat that much, believe her instead of thinking she is just piling away the goodies or how else could she be so fat. Get support by networking with other professionals from the various discipline areas who are working with this paradigm. Meet with those folks in your area informally, and reach out to others. Be PRO-ACTIVE. Let others know how you feel by organizing training for this paradigm. It takes VIGILANCE with ourselves and others to stay on track because we are constantly bombarded with the other message. And most of all, don't lose your sense of humor about it. Lighten up and laugh at yourself and the culture every now and again.

Terry W., Psy.D., Psychologist, Fresno, California

What types of clients are best suited for a nondiet approach?

Clients that seem more amenable to this approach are those who have personally experienced either the failure of yo-yo dieting, the obsessions and psychic pain of struggling with an eating disorder, or the health consequences of repeated weight loss dieting or an eating disorder.

I think without a widespread prevention program to promote acceptance of body diversity at an early age it is harder to reach adolescents and college age women who are under so much pressure to be thin--and who often aren't yet conscious of the consequences of the thinness ideal and repeated efforts to lose weight.

How do you work with other professionals/colleagues who may not be comfortable with a nondiet approach?

Nonjudgmental education.

What words of wisdom do you have for those who are beginning to explore a nondiet paradigm?

Keep an open mind! This is a paradigm shift that flies in the face of most of the messages we get today about body, beauty, and weight.

6

HUNGERWORK: Promote Joyful and Healthful Eating

> *For the most part, women with eating problems have spent a lifetime abdicating control of what they eat and being discouraged from discovering what their preferences or dislikes are. They are unaware that different foods can give them many possible sensations, that their moods or bodily states prefer various foods at different times. Food groups are seen as good or bad, fattening or not, high or low-calorie; women often have almost no clue beyond these highly charged notions about how to nourish their hungry bodies in a sensually satisfying way (1).*

Moving Away From Diets provides a framework for you and your clients to facilitate a path to self-care. Modification of eating style can be a vital health enhancing opportunity on this path. In order to facilitate these changes and promote a normal (2), nourishing eating style, clients must:

- reconnect with internal cues of hunger and satiety,
- work on accepting their natural size and shape,
- make food choices in a nonrestrained environment,
- be provided with pertinent nutrition information in a manner free of moralization.

A common misconception of the nondiet approach is that by neutralizing food and eating unrestrained in response to internal cues, nutrition and health axioms are no longer needed. On the contrary, nutrition information is most valuable and affirming in this exact context. Providing nutrition information for clients in the nondiet paradigm involves blending their food experiences and discoveries with what is known about food and its impact on health.

Joyful eating and healthful eating go hand in hand. Both will blossom in a neutral, nonjudgmental setting. Joyful eating primarily stems from being free to explore and experiment with food, recognizing the sensual aspects of the food experience. Healthful eating primarily stems from identifying, interpreting, and meeting physical needs. Eating attuned to internal cues guides not only quantity, but also the variety of food selected. Clients report that over time, staying attuned to their internal cues results in a more healthful eating style, and inseparably, a more pleasurable experience.

MEDICAL NUTRITION THERAPY

"Medical nutrition therapy involves the assessment of the nutritional status of patients with a condition, illness, or injury that puts them at risk. This includes review and analysis of medical and diet history, laboratory values, and anthropometric measurement. Based on the assessment, nutrition modalities most appropriate to manage the condition or treat the illness or injury are chosen, and include the following:

- Diet modification and counseling leading to the development of a personal diet plan to achieve nutritional goals and desired health outcomes.
- Specialized nutrition therapies including supplementation with medical foods for those unable to obtain adequate nutrients through food intake only; enteral nutrition delivered via tube feeding into the gastrointestinal tract for those unable to ingest or digest food; and parenteral nutrition delivered via intravenous infusion for those unable to absorb nutrients (3)."

Moving Away From Diets is fundamentally compatible with The American Dietetic Association's above definition of medical nutrition therapy. Research tells us dieting and restrained eating are often ineffective in the long term. HungerWork helps individuals break away from restrained eating that promotes or results in unsatisfying eating styles and accompanying negative psychological and physiological side effects (4,5).

By promoting self-acceptance and size acceptance, individuals come to recognize they are entitled and uniquely qualified to identify and satisfy their own needs for food. This process shifts the locus of control from external to internal. In this context individuals can explore modifying their food intake without the threat of deprivation. By working through the three facets of HungerWork, a truly personal eating style emerges that considers clients' nutritional goals, medical conditions, and desired health outcomes.

> *I used to have some peculiar attitudes about food. I never ate sandwiches because doing so implied I was entitled to eat a whole serving of something. I picked at food and was picky about food. I needed every calorie to go beyond satisfaction. When I ate for volume, I felt unsatisfied. When I ate for satisfaction, I missed the volume. I believed if I ate for both I'd start bingeing and gaining weight. I have since rediscovered the sensual aspects of food. I am no longer picky, but selective. I want quality. I am not only entitled to eat a sandwich, I want the best sandwich I can make. I want colors, flavors, textures, health. I want all that food can uniquely provide.*
>
> *T.K., Restaurateur, Pasadena, CA*

ASSESSING CLIENT READINESS FOR QUALITY OF INTAKE WORK

The way in which food is sensed and processed by the biological system generates neural and humoral signals, which are used to control appetite. It follows that any self-imposed or externally applied reduction in the food supply, creating a calorific deficit, will weaken the satiating power of food. One consequence of this will be the failure of food to suppress hunger adequately (the biological drive) (6).

Advertisements propagate that food has the power to keep us centered, provide passion, draw families together, and even entice a love interest. Food advertisements and food attitudes contain very confusing messages, especially for young women when they are combined with the plethora of beauty myths and diet advertisements. By eating in a restrained manner, individuals unknowingly create a situation where they are longing (physically or psychologically) for chocolate chip cookies. Crashing through their desire is the warning... "Danger, danger, danger...don't eat any because they are fattening!" The individual who disregards the warning, and eats the cookies then feels incredibly guilty and scared. These feelings need to be expressed. *Food must be neutralized and eating unrestrained before the individual can be fully receptive to nutrition information.*

> *Providing nutrition information can worsen problematic eating if the health care provider uses (or the client perceives) a moralistic framework about type or amount of food.*

Another barrier to accepting nutrition information is expecting food to do more than abate hunger and satisfy appetite. The mere fact that clients cannot make food take problems away or emotional emptiness, prompts and perpetuates an "out of control" feeling. Eventually resentment builds up towards the food because it does not do what they hoped, or thought food promised to do.

Inviting a client to explore foods and look more closely at their food history, can be likened to leading the criminal back to the scene of the crime or the victim back to the location of the assault or intrusion. Many restrained eaters see themselves as a criminal (guilty of horrific food crimes) or a victim of intrusion or assault (food being the perpetrator or the attacker).

By keeping rigid rules, clients believe they are protecting themselves from committing food crimes, while keeping the perpetrator out. It is actually an attempt to assert themselves and set boundaries. However, the consequences and side effects are costly. They never feel at peace with food, never let their guard down, constantly declare themselves guilty or weak. The health care provider that can understand this depth of pain and recrimination will be able to gently challenge and support the client in exploring food.

In light of these distorted, painful histories with food, many clients gain the most benefit from promoting joyful and healthful eating after they have made considerable progress in recovering from their deprivation-driven eating and emotional, compulsive eating. (See chapters three, four, and five.) "Considerable progress" is meant to be subjective. Clients that have worked on the earlier HungerWork facets are the most freed and receptive to enhancing their pleasure and health through food.

> *Over time with proper care, bodily sensations become organized, knowable, alive, personal, and even pleasurable...If the infant has a need, it can be understood and met; pleasure then accrues to both parts of the experience, the need itself and the response (1).*

INTRODUCING JOYFUL AND HEALTHFUL EATING TO A CLIENT

Following are two suggestions for promoting joyful and healthful eating to clients individually or in groups. You can vary the depth and intensity of the discussions depending on the readiness of your clients.

Eating Style Fantasy

In a group setting or individually, encourage clients to fantasize and describe how they would like their eating style to be and what they hope food could do for them. Very often, clients cannot do this without including their idealized body shape or size in the discussion. This brings up the familiar dilemma, "If I'm satisfied with food, I'll gain an incredible amount of weight. If I'm satisfied with my weight, I won't be able to eat any food." If this happens, explore this perception. Because of the psychological and physiological side effects of restrained eating, it is very difficult for these clients to imagine a satisfying eating style being compatible with a stable, natural weight.

This fantasy exercise may also be difficult because clients have a tendency to avoid talking about foods they believe they "shouldn't" eat, even though they may often think about these foods secretively or shamefully. It helps the client end the secrecy and shame if they can talk about foods and food behaviors in a trustworthy, nonjudgmental environment. Nurturing open, sensitive dialogue through the difficult aspects of this exercise promotes acceptance and bonding within a group. Whenever the health care provider models client acceptance, clients learn more about self-acceptance.

Inviting Food Over for Dinner

Put out a food tray with an average day's food supply for one person. Choose foods that may be viewed as "good" or "diet" foods and some that may be viewed as "fattening" or "bad." Include foods that are attractive, colorful, aromatic. Solicit responses and reactions from group members. Common responses are:

"It looks like a lot of food."

"It looks like a diet."

"What if I don't want to eat that? Do I have to?"

"I could never eat that much, is that what we're supposed to eat?"

"I'm not comfortable with food being here tonight."

"Do we get to eat it?"

"What if someone takes the thing I want?"

"I don't want to eat in front of anyone."

Welcome and affirm all reactions. Acknowledge that it is interesting how varied feelings are about food. Eat the food together. If a group member does not want to eat, or prefers to take his or her portion home, affirm the right to make food decisions on his or her own. This is especially effective with a psychotherapist present. Consider including, if appropriate, the nutritional breakdown of the food, such as: calories, protein, fat, calcium, iron, fiber, 5 a-day, etc. A group that has worked extensively on neutralizing food (removing the "good" and "bad" food labels) will be more receptive to nutritional information about food. A group that is just beginning to neutralize food will likely be resistant to nutrition information. They may even feel restricted from foods not on the tray or obligated to include the foods on display into their eating style.

EXPERIMENTING WITH THE MEAL MIX TO FIND JOY AND HEALTH

> *Oh, wow, I finally get it. The only bad food is the moldy stuff in the back of my refrigerator!*
>
> A moment of enlightenment...
> Laurice B., Administrator, Glendale, California

Keep in mind there is no good food or bad food, except, perhaps in describing the sanitation or freshness of food. Meal mix is a term discussed earlier that refers to the proportion of fats, proteins (animal and vegetable), carbohydrates (simple and complex), and fiber (soluble and insoluble) in a meal or snack. Meal mix also considers the impact caffeine, alcohol, artificial sweeteners, and fat substitutes have on hunger, fullness, satiety, and laboratory values. (See Alexis' Food Journal and discussion on pages 54 and 55.) The purposes of working with the meal mix are to:

- Discover clients' preferred ratio of protein, fat, carbohydrate, and fiber in each snack or meal.
- Relay pertinent nutrition guidance and information based on clients' personal goals, health status and their preferred eating style without using moralized terms.
- Equip clients with experience and knowledge so they can choose foods that match their internal cues, expectations, and health goals, time after time.

Freedom to Experiment With Food

In order for clients to discover their preferred meal mix, they need to become aware of how food feels after eating it, and its impact on their health and sense of well-being. For example, if clients discover that some foods make them groggy if eaten at lunch, while other foods are energizing, they move closer to being able to choose foods to elicit the response and benefits they want. Most restrained eaters do not allow themselves to freely experiment with food. In order for them to know what they want, and what satisfies them, they need to be given the opportunity and support to explore.

Satisfying Senses Through Meal Mix

All five senses play exciting roles as clients experiment. Invite them to picture (or have available in a session) the spectacular rainbow of red, yellow, orange, green, and purple bell peppers. Take in the wafting aroma of fresh gingerbread cooling on the counter. Hear the crisp crunch upon biting into a chilled, juicy pippin apple or the music of silverware tapping a dish. Watch children eat; they love exploring food with their hands as they immerse themselves in the experience, literally and figuratively! And finally, cherish the flavor of a New York style cheesecake with fresh raspberries on top. In the experimental phase, encourage clients to ask themselves such questions as:

Will this food give me vitality, health, and energy?

How did I feel last time I ate this food?

Am I enjoying this food as much now as when I took my first few bites?

Is the amount I have on my plate going to satisfy me?

If it's not enough, can I get more now, or will I be able to get some again tomorrow?

These are very challenging, and sometimes overwhelming questions for clients to ask themselves. Meet clients where they are and set the pace accordingly.

TREATMENT STRATEGIES AND TECHNIQUES FOR DISCOVERING PLEASURE AND HEALTH

Guiding clients in making healthful, informed food choices involves spending time exploring the **subjective** realm to experience joyful eating and the **objective** realm to incorporate healthful eating (such as, protein requirements and blood glucose values). Following are five tools and techniques you can use to help your clients develop a joyful, healthful eating style.

Use a Food/Feelings Journal

The Food Journal, Figure 4-A on page 51, is a visual display of both the subjective realm (attitudes, preferences, satiety) and the objective realm (fiber intake, calcium sources, frequency of meals). It is helpful to see the contrast between a client's perception of fullness, what was consumed, and the resulting satisfaction. Often, a client will eat to a greater degree of fullness if the meal is not satisfying. As if to say, "If I'm not getting the quality I want, I'll have to get quantity." Or, "I've eaten junky food all day, why stop now?" Although any meal pattern guide can be used, including the Pyramid, *this food journal is set up to coordinate with the* **Core Minimum Daily Food Choice Guide,** Figure 6-A (7). *Note:* protein units are interchangeable.

Reviewing food/feelings journals from weeks past can provide evidence of progress. Clients benefit from regular reinforcement from the health care provider. Identify what has changed. Encourage them in behaviors, perspective shifts and activities that are in line with their personal goals. This helps clients learn how to track their progress in the nondiet paradigm so they can recognize success (8). Continually ask clients if the foods they are selecting are enjoyable, satisfying, and energizing.

Food/feelings journals can help clients identify and understand why they start and stop eating. They may start eating for physical reasons (hunger) and stop for non-physical reasons (guilt, interruption, food is gone). Or, they may start for emotional reasons (needing comfort) and stop for physical reasons (fullness or sleepiness). A healthful eating style, psychologically and physically, starts and stops most of the time from physical hunger and satiety cues.

Rather than use the terms, "healthy/ unhealthy," "good/ bad," or even, "good/ not so good," I have been using the terms "supportive/ non-supportive." I do not determine the foods that go into these categories, the client does. My goal is that, over time, they will see what foods support their health/recovery, and what foods do not. Amy Brewer, RD, Memphis, TN

Figure 6-A Core Minimum Daily Food Choice Guide

THE CORE MINIMUM

DAILY FOOD GROUPS

PRIMARY PROTEIN SOURCE

DAIRY PROTEINS

4 units minimum *

-- 1 c milk **
-- 1/2 c yogurt **
-- 1/4 c cottage cheese
-- 2 Tbsp grated parmesan cheese
-- 1 oz cheese
-- 1 oz ricotta cheese
-- 1/4 c dry milk, instant

BEAN / MEAT PROTEINS

4 units minimum

-- 1 oz chicken, turkey, fish, meat
-- 2 oz shrimp, scallops, crab, lobster, clams
-- 1/4 c tuna, chicken
-- 1/2 c cooked beans (legumes)
-- 3 oz tofu
-- 2 egg whites
-- 1 whole egg
-- 2 rounded Tbsp peanut butter

PRIMARY COMPLEX CARBOHYDRATE SOURCES

FRUITS AND VEGETABLES

5 units minimum

-- average serving fruit (medium apple,
   banana, orange, grapefruit half)
-- 1/4 any melon (8" size)
-- 1 c melon
-- 1/2 c fruit or vegetable juice
-- 1/2 c sliced fruit (grapes, pineapple, etc.)
-- 1/4 c dried fruit
-- 1/2 c cooked vegetables
-- 1 c raw vegetables

GRAINS (STARCHES)

9 units minimum

-- 1 slice bread
-- 1/2 bagel, 1/2 large pita, 1/2 hamburger bun,
   1/2 english muffin
-- 1/2 c cooked cereal
-- 1/2 c rice, 1/2 c pasta
-- 1 oz ready-to-eat breakfast cereal (~1/2 c)
-- 1 small roll, biscuit, or muffin
-- 5 to 6 small crackers
-- 2 rice cakes
-- 1/2 medium potato
-- 1/2 c green peas or corn

OTHERS

Use to round out meals and meet energy
requirements

-- Fats - oils, butter, margarine, mayonnaise,
   bacon, olives
-- Sweets - sugar, honey, jam, syrup, jelly,
   candy, sugared gum
-- Desserts - cake, cookies, donuts, pastries,
   pies
-- Beverages (sugar - based)
-- Et Cetera !

* 6 units minimum of dairy protein for
  pregnant/breastfeeding women and teens

**best calcium source

YOUR MINIMUM PLAN IS:

Milk Protein	B/M Protein	Fruit/ Veg	Grain	Others

Use the Hunger Scale

Through tracking internal cues on the Hunger Scale, clients learn to identify their bodies' physical cues in various stages of hunger, fullness, and satiety. Through using the principles in this chapter, you affirm their experience and interpretation of these cues by explaining the relevant physiological and nutritional principles. In turn, clients are able to incorporate sound, pertinent nutrition information, internal cues, and desired outcomes into their food decisions. The following discussion between Jayne and her health care provider, Terri, illustrates this identification, affirmation, and learning process:

Jayne: I'm hungry at breakfast and lunch but I'm having trouble getting hungry enough at dinner time to eat with my family. I've even cut out my afternoon cookies hoping that would help. Now all I buy on my break is an iced cafe latte and I'm still not as hungry as I'd like to be by dinner at 5:30 p.m. I feel pretty discouraged. I guess I'll just have to eat later, alone, without the company of my family.

Terri: It makes sense, Jayne that you may not get hungry by dinnertime on days that you substitute the latte for the cookies. You've made lattes at home before. What's in a latte that might keep you from getting hungry by 5:30 p.m.?

Jayne: Well, there's milk and sugar in it. Both have calories. But a latte isn't food, it's a drink.

Terri: Your body "reads" it as food. Even though the latte is mostly water, those calories are in the form of protein, fat, and carbohydrates. Your latte is also a source of calcium with nearly 10 ounces of low fat milk in it. Did you know yogurt has these same nutrients in similar proportions, just less water?

Jayne: So, that's why the latte satisfies my slight hunger in the late afternoon, and I don't get hungry again until about 6:30 p.m. I wonder if eating a yogurt would make me feel the same. Maybe if I have half a cup of yogurt, one cookie, or the small latte I can get through the late afternoon AND be hungry by 5:30 p.m. I'd like to try it.

Terri: I'm looking forward to hearing about your discoveries, Jayne, you are our data gatherer, so be sure to remain judgment-free this week. You will discover so much more about yourself by doing so. Have fun!

Use the Food Guide Pyramid

A nonjudgmental environment is essential in order for you and clients to assess nutritional adequacy together. For some clients, just the suggestion of categorizing food into nutritional food groups triggers dieting memories. They may suddenly begin criticizing their food choices or themselves for not "eating right." They may become defensive of what they have eaten. They may feel angry with you or resentful. Help your clients express these feelings and the resulting self-talk. Helping them understand what triggers the old thoughts and feelings is instrumental in shifting back to the nondiet paradigm.

The Food Guide Pyramid, Figure 6-B, features average serving sizes and nutrient equivalents rather than caloric equivalents. Review the pyramid with clients explaining the basic food groups. You can also use the Core Minimum Daily Food Choice Guide, Figure 6-A, for clients that need to see some suggested serving sizes. Include the following points:

❖ Confirm with the client that not all foods in each group have the same number of calories. They will know this and will want to make sure you do, too!

❖ Let them know from a nutritional standpoint, the foods in each group are interchangeable. The goal is to expand choices, focus less on calories and more on natural, relaxed eating. Some clients have a great need to know exact calories in order to eat. It is important to meet clients where they are with the goal for them to move away from calorie counting.

❖ Reinforce the Food Guide Pyramid with the Food Journal. In the squares at the bottom of the journal clients can total their intake at the end of the day or they can preset their intake goal for the day. It is important that clients not view this goal as a diet; only as a nutritional guide for enhancing their health.

Mini Case Study

Peggy just started a new job and needs to leave her house in the mornings by 6:30. She discovered she is not hungry for breakfast until about 9:00 a.m. Due to her commute, she does not arrive home at night until 7:00 p.m. Knowing her body's needs and hunger patterns she decides to bring breakfast, lunch, and snacks from home. Peggy feels her best if she can stay between 2 and 7 on the Hunger Scale (0-10). She also knows her body asks for about 1,800-2,300 calories a day and by 5:00 p.m. she needs to have eaten about three quarters of her food for the day. Peggy enjoys some packaged, frozen foods because of their convenience and tastes. With the use of food labels, Peggy can find a multitude of foods to pack for breakfast, lunch, and snacks, add up the calories (and protein) to assure she has ample provisions for the day. (Her old diet view was to check food labels to find foods lowest in calories and fat, highest in volume.)

Dispelling food myths

Once we decide to give food and its preparation and enjoyment, some time and what might occasionally be called reverence, we may find that good food and good-for-you food are more likely to come from deep in the past from ancient cultures and traditions that...found their inspiration close to the land (9).

Often restrained eaters retain myths and misunderstandings from their diet histories. Gently dispelling food myths is one important aspect of HungerWork. Numerous opportunities arise, but the key to being effective is continually maintaining a nonjudgmental, open, explorative tone. Jayne presents a common misconception to her dietitian, Terri:

Jayne: I don't overeat every day. I do have some good days. For instance, my ideal day is having black coffee and a plain bagel for breakfast followed by pasta with marinara sauce and iced tea for lunch. It seems like the less I eat in the morning the better. I get so discouraged though. I feel fine until hunger hits me like a truck in the afternoon.

Terri: Bodies are fascinating! Did you know that bodies use protein for muscle repair, wound healing, immune system function, enzymes and hormones? In addition, it is common to find that having protein at breakfast or lunch brings on a more gradual sense of hunger as the day progresses. If this were the case for you, Jayne, would that be helpful?"

Jayne: I guess so. I don't want to overeat at breakfast, but I suppose if it helps me feel better in the afternoon that might be a fair trade-off. I could try it one or two days this week and see how it goes.

Terri: I'll be interested in what you find out about yourself.

Whether Jayne has a satisfying or unsatisfying experience, the dietitian affirms why it went the way it did. The next step is to ask Jayne how the information she just gathered about her body is useful. (In addition to including protein, Jayne may need to repeat the same experiment with more calories, fat, and fiber.) If Jayne is unsure of other protein sources, a fun, educational opportunity presents itself to put the spotlight on the pleasures of food...especially using creative, dynamic, descriptive words such as, succulent, fresh, juicy, ripe.

Figure 6-C Food Guide Pyramid

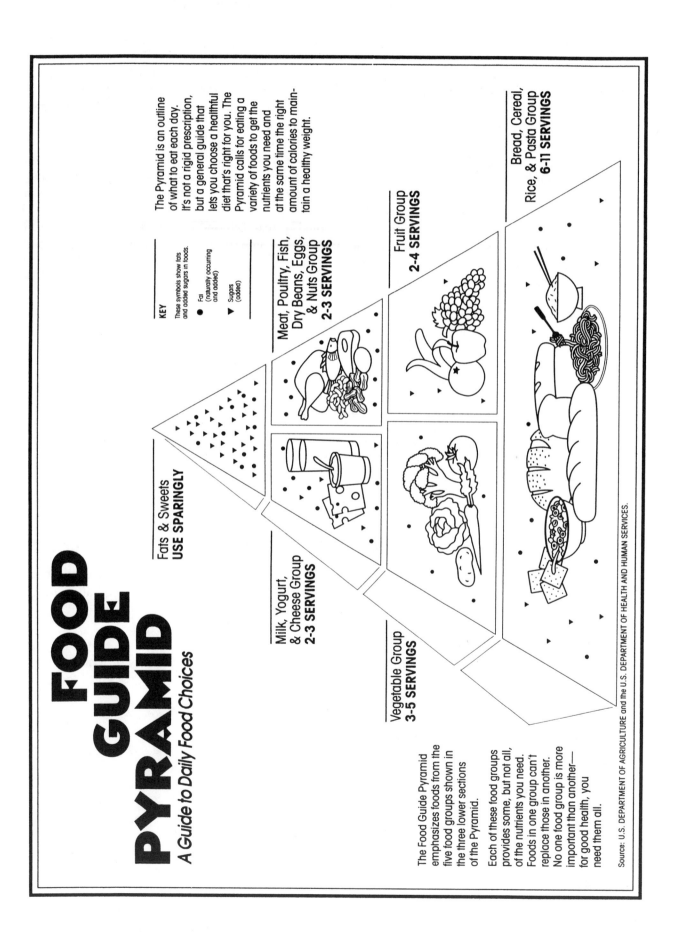

FOOD GUIDE PYRAMID
A Guide to Daily Food Choices

The Food Guide Pyramid emphasizes foods from the five food groups shown in the three lower sections of the Pyramid.

Each of these food groups provides some, but not all, of the nutrients you need. Foods in one group can't replace those in another. No one food group is more important than another—for good health, you need them all.

Fats & Sweets
USE SPARINGLY

KEY
These symbols show fats and added sugars in foods.
● Fat (naturally occurring and added)
▼ Sugars (added)

The Pyramid is an outline of what to eat each day. It's not a rigid prescription, but a general guide that lets you choose a healthful diet that's right for you. The Pyramid calls for eating a variety of foods to get the nutrients you need and at the same time the right amount of calories to maintain a healthy weight.

Milk, Yogurt, & Cheese Group
2-3 SERVINGS

Meat, Poultry, Fish, Dry Beans, Eggs, & Nuts Group
2-3 SERVINGS

Vegetable Group
3-5 SERVINGS

Fruit Group
2-4 SERVINGS

Bread, Cereal, Rice, & Pasta Group
6-11 SERVINGS

Source: U.S. DEPARTMENT OF AGRICULTURE and the U.S. DEPARTMENT OF HEALTH AND HUMAN SERVICES.

Using Food Labels to Expand Choices

Nutrition information on food labels helps clients become familiar with food composition as it relates to their preferred meal mix.

For example, Robert has diabetes. Through experimentation, he is just discovering a certain quantity of carbohydrates cause blood glucose to remain above his preferred level following the meal. Determining the amount of carbohydrate he takes in when his subsequent blood glucose values are in his desired range comes from experimenting with the meal. He can also learn how carbohydrates influence his glucose levels differently depending on the amount of protein, fats, and complex or simple carbohydrates he consumes in that same meal (10).

He is learning that he feels satisfied from a meal that contains more carbohydrates than he thought he was "supposed" to have. Considering the importance of being satisfied, Robert and his health care provider can now expand his choices by identifying additional foods from reading the nutrition label together that contain similar amounts of carbohydrates. This also assures him greater satisfaction from the eating experience.

Robert has a few options to accommodate his preferred carbohydrate intake: he can increase his insulin dosage (or oral medication) or he can experiment with adjusting the time and duration of his physical activity (if he is so inclined), or a combination of these two. The goal is to manage blood glucose based on his preferred eating style.

Note: Many clients believe if their blood glucose level goes too high, they cannot eat the "culprit" food. The nondiet approach directs the client back to the eating event and asks the following questions:

> Was I hungry?
> Did I stop eating when I was comfortably full?
> Did I eat what I wanted?
> Did I feel nourished and satisfied after the meal?

If the client answers "yes" to these questions, review how to adjust insulin (or medication) to that meal mix, rather than restrict the amount based on blood glucose response. With "no" type responses, support them in exploring hunger, satiety, and discriminating between emotional eating and physically-connected eating.

IN SEARCH OF SATIETY

> *Nothing is so effective in keeping one young and full of lust as a discriminating palate thoroughly satisfied at least once a day.* Angelo Pellegrini (9)

Chapters three, four, and five discuss helping clients identify and respond to various eating cues. Likewise, you can play a significant role in helping clients attain satisfaction from food. Following are suggested techniques:

Define Satisfaction

Assist clients in defining their experience of feeling satisfied versus full. Identify patterns. Is there a higher level of satisfaction from eating whole or fresh foods versus processed, packaged foods? Or is it the other way around?

Identify Barriers to Satisfaction

Some clients do not grocery shop as needed. They view fresh food as "a hassle to prepare or a waste of money because it goes bad." They eat haphazardly. They are not satisfied nor do they see the value in being satisfied. They may eat fast food frequently or all food fast. They may exhibit other inattentive eating behaviors. Explore these behaviors as perhaps attempts to cut off from pleasurable, sensual experiences, avoid needs identification, and prohibit self-gratification. (Clients' deeper issues may also need to be processed with a mental health professional.)

Invest in Satisfaction
Encourage clients to get involved in shopping, planning, and preparation. If their life responsibilities seem overwhelming, they may be able to shop and prepare only one meal in a week. It could be extremely helpful if session time is spent on meal planning. Investing themselves in selecting, gathering, and preparing the meal will enhance their experience and result in greater satisfaction. The goal is to involve them as much as possible in their food experience.

APPRECIATING THE FULL EXPERIENCE
Heighten a client's awareness of the full food experience using the acronym A.F.T.E.R.
   A=appearance F=flavor T=temperature/texture E=experience R=results (11).

A: Is the **appearance** enticing? Are the colors pleasing and varied? Are shapes or designs noticeable, such as the starburst design inside a kiwi fruit? Is the table set attractively? Is there something to add to enhance the ambiance, such as candles or eating outdoors? Does the presentation match expectations?

F: Notice the **flavors** each food contributes and how they blend together. Is there one that is especially pleasing? Flavors are enhanced by aroma. Notice aroma while the food is being prepared. With eyes closed take in the scents of fresh peaches, and other favorites. Experiment with salty, sour, sweet, and bitter on the taste buds. To prevent deprivation, make plans to have pleasurable foods again, soon.

T: Is the food at the desirable **temperature**? If not, would it enhance the experience to correct it? If so, take the time to do it. Are there **temperature** and **texture** combinations that add interest, such as chicken fresh off the grill laid on a bed of chilled salad greens? Key in on the textures. Do the foods satisfy the need to chew? Notice the various textures on the plate. Focus on the feeling of smooth foods in the mouth contrasted with crunchy.

E: Was the overall **experience** enjoyable? What kinds of emotions were experienced? Was the ambiance pleasing? Were there sounds of nature, music, happy voices, laughter? Was the environment conducive to experiencing the food? Were there distractions that could be avoided next time? Did the environment make it difficult to stay in touch with internal signals of satiety or fullness? If so, make a note for next time. What aspects of the experience could be replicated next time?

R: **Results** of the meal are a vital aspect of this exercise and frequently the most overlooked. What were the results of the meal experience? Was the desired fullness or satiety level reached? Did the client feel energized or relaxed? Did the client end the meal feeling nurtured, encouraged, joyful, guilt-free? Finally, did the food sustain the client until the next meal? What adjustments can be made to enhance the next eating experience?

As clients pay greater attention to some or all of these aspects of the eating experience, they begin to identify the degree they are satisfied or unsatisfied. After some time, clients will be able to eat when physically hungry and stop at a comfortable level of fullness. Until they can attend to appetite and satiation, many clients continue feeling unsatisfied or bored with food, and do not know why.

Being satisfied at every meal or snack is unrealistic for most busy lifestyles. Sometimes hunger is abated, but the appetite is not satisfied. These are occasions when foods available are unappealing to the individual at that time, but the intensifying hunger requires them to eat purely for fuel. This is a part of normal eating and must be accepted in order for clients to be content with their food relationship.

SUMMARY OF PROMOTING JOYFUL, HEALTHFUL EATING
The health care provider's role is two-fold.

1. Guiding the client in nonrestrained eating to enhance the biochemical mechanisms involved in satiety (12,13).
2. Guiding clients to a psychologically healthful relationship with food. To the degree clients are free to fully experience their food, is the degree to which they have an opportunity to be satiated.

MOVING AWAY FROM MEDICAL DIETS AND NUTRITION-SENSITIVE DISEASES

Note: Diabetes is used predominantly in this section to illustrate how to apply HungerWork, however, many other nutrition-sensitive diseases and chronic illnesses can use the approach: hyperlipidemias, hypertension, renal failure, gastrointestinal disorders, and food allergies or sensitivities.

Understandably, clients with nutrition-sensitive diseases go through a transition period when they shift to a physically-connected eating style. Diabetes is the most common example. Usually, clients' medication (insulin or oral agents) requires adjustment throughout the transition as they experiment with food. Hence, the need for frequent self-monitoring of blood glucose for feedback.

Consider clients' age, mental and physical stability, other health risks, personal support, and how long they can or will work on making the change. Hold firm to the motto "Do no harm."

Occasionally, clients are not good candidates for HungerWork. Sometimes clients with critical mental or physical illness benefit by making minimal, gradual or externally-directed changes, rather than going through the process of a paradigm shift in their eating style. Also, some clients' status pose a high risk such as an insulin-dependent individual with an eating disorder, who is unwilling to self-monitor blood glucose. Working with these clients toward openness and eventually a commitment to self-monitor blood glucose can move them out of the high risk category. Usually, a treatment team approach is most effective (physician, dietitian, and mental health professional).

Facilitating a Perspective Shift in Clients With Nutrition-Sensitive Diseases
Treatment strategies and techniques:

Lift moralization off of food
In light of clients' conditions or diseases, reframe (help them think differently about) "good and bad" food.

For example, Kelly is seeing a dietitian for the first time, just having been informed by her nephrologist that she needs to reduce her protein intake to less than 60 grams a day:
Dietitian: "Kelly, protein is not a "bad" food. Protein is a life-sustaining nutrient. We will work together to discover the amount you naturally seem to want, the amount your body can tolerate, and the amount you need for sustenance."

Not only does this remove the "good and bad" food categories, it also provides an educational sound bite (protein is a life-sustaining nutrient). Choosing terminology within a nonjudgmental framework facilitates a paradigm shift.

Present fundamentals of the condition in a nonjudgmental way
This may be the first time clients learn about their condition and its physiology without blaming themselves or feeling criticized. Help clients identify philosophies or self-management skills from their past they would like to integrate into their lifestyles now. Encourage clients to bring the positive aspects of their past with them, and begin letting go of painful or frightening experiences, self-talk and knowledge that are harmful or inaccurate. Sometimes this process may require switching to or adding an additional health care provider that is familiar with the nondiet approach.

Help clients reframe (think differently about) lab values
Move blood glucose values into a neutral framework. Equate blood glucose monitoring and resultant

levels with taking their temperature with a thermometer. It is neither good nor bad; but an indicator of what is happening inside their body. Sometimes clients do not want to test, "I don't want to see numbers that show how bad I feel." Explore from the perspective that reality can be painful; it is understandable they would put up a defense in the form of resistance. Discuss how this defense helps them and limits them. Through expressing their fears and other feelings, they may be able to reframe glucose monitoring as a way to learn about their body and what it needs.

Encourage clients to accept their bodies

Many clients with nutrition-sensitive diseases have difficulty accepting their bodies and may not be attentive or responsive to their bodies' needs. They may believe their bodies are "bad" or "broken." Joan M. Lyman, MS, MFCC is a therapist who specializes in the psychosocial aspects of chronic diseases and has had diabetes for 41 years. She explains, *"Shortly after comprehending the magnitude of the medical diagnosis, the client may begin to feel defective. Feeling defective breeds shame. The shame is so painful, they move into denial. Often the client fears, 'What will go wrong next? I can't trust my body. It doesn't work right. I'm a bad person.' This sense of being defective leads to isolation from people in their life. They may also think, 'My partner is getting a raw deal. I'm a burden to my partner.' This self-talk creates another barrier to intimacy and connection. An end result can be a client who is disconnected from his or her body, self, family, and friends (15)."*

Treatment team members may be the only people these clients are connected to, especially regarding their disease. Modeling acceptance, support, and shared responsibility in a nonjudgmental atmosphere can facilitate reconnection for clients to themselves, as well as to family and friends.

The following case study incorporates treatment strategies and techniques from HungerWork. Note the interlacing of promoting both joyful and healthful eating.

Case Study
Andy

At his recent physical exam, Andy's physician informed him that his cholesterol level was high. He also said intake of saturated fat in certain quantities may be elevating his serum cholesterol levels, increasing his risk for heart disease. The physician referred him to a dietitian for advice. Knowing butter is a source of saturated fat, and assuming the dietitian would say the same, Andy decided butter was a "bad" food and has been trying to avoid it whenever possible. He really enjoys butter, and occasionally has indulged out of "weakness." At these times, he has felt guilty and worried about his health.

In his first session with the dietitian, Andy hears her say something surprising, "Before you cross butter permanently off your shopping list, how would you feel about taking a closer look at butter?" Andy answers, "Yes," with a note of curiosity and hope in his voice.

He begins exploring the **subjective** realm of his food preferences with the guidance of the dietitian. He is asked to put butter on some food in the next week when he feels the desire. This begins the process of neutralizing butter while he identifies when he has a desire for butter. When he eats the butter the dietitian suggests he asks himself the following questions,

Is it as satisfying as I expected?

Was I actually desiring butter, or would another source of fat or condiment be as satisfying or more so?

In what ways is the taste and mouth feel of butter the same or different as other fats?

Including the **objective** realm means adding to Andy's nutrition knowledge about fats in a nonjudgmental way, such as:

Dietary fats have health and sensory enhancing attributes.

Healthy bodies require dietary fats for optimal health.

Fats enhance the aromas, tastes, and textures of foods.

Other fats have similar attributes with lower levels of saturated fat than butter.

Eating some fat in a meal may enhance satiety value of the meal and postpone the onset
of subsequent hunger (14,15).

Some individuals find their serum cholesterol level elevates when they consume certain
quantities of saturated fats.

Some reduction in these saturated fats, while maintaining some mono- and
polyunsaturated fats in an eating style may help reduce serum cholesterol.

Andy returns the next week with the data he gathered from experimenting with butter. He recognizes there were times he was very satisfied with butter and times he could have gone without it.

His next project is to explore other sources of fats (peanut butter, olive oil, avocado). This will prove to be a fun adventure! Furthermore, he certainly does not have to do it alone, unless he chooses to. The dietitian suggests various ways he can experiment. They could taste test different fats during their next session, such as olive oil and garlic on French bread. Or, Andy could experiment with a culinary or gourmet group, nondiet support group, or join a friend at a restaurant. Any of these can add to the enjoyment of his meal.

Andy may discover he enjoys other healthful fats. He may gradually open up to new tastes and textures in familiar foods but with more health enhancing fats. By being guided into this subjective realm, he will experience blending appetite and knowledge together as he makes food choices. Andy may also wish he had joined a culinary appreciation group sooner!

Identifying and Healing Problematic Self-Management Styles (As Applied to Diabetes)

For patients with diabetes, an important goal in the effort to move toward health is to attain the best possible metabolic control. Equally desirable, however, is for patients to reach and control the necessary intrinsic resources and to become engaged in treating their own disease to a sufficient extent to achieve a feeling of well-being (12).

In response to the results of the DCCT (Diabetes Control and Complications Trial [16]), many clients with diabetes (IDDM and NIDDM) are learning how to maintain tighter control of their blood glucose levels through intensive insulin therapy. The results of the trial show this dramatically reduces risks of long-term complications (i.e. kidney failure, visual impairment, nerve damage). These results are empowering for individuals as they can influence their sense of well-being and the quality of their health over the long run (17,18).

Some clients with diabetes, however, hear this information in such a way that they abdicate their personal power. This "power shift" results in feeling restricted and controlled. If these clients eat outside their physical cues or allow their blood glucose levels to go outside the recommended range for tight control (19), they feel guilt, anger, and resentment...they feel trapped. In order for clients to experience a sense of well-being, the psychosocial issues around their diabetes need to be explored.

Therefore, gently exploring their motivations for maintaining tight control and expected outcome is imperative. What may be revealed is a coping strategy likened to a dieter's mentality. This mentality is actually fostered by a perspective that authority and direction come primarily from outside the individual (an external locus of control). The locus of control remains external by strategies perceived as obligations, such as, calorie counting, exchange groups, carbohydrate counting, moralizing blood glucose levels as "good and bad," or viewing themselves as "good or bad."

Clients may also hide their preoccupation with thinness by using their condition to justify food restriction and the pursuit of thinness. The diet mentality is the client's chosen method of "doing the right thing" or maintaining a sense of control. Paradoxically, the locus of control remains outside of them, rather than moving inward (20,21).

Point of Clarification: This is *not* to say managing blood glucose levels through a counting or tracking method is inappropriate. The concepts in *Moving Away From Diets* facilitate internally-motivated and internally-directed self-care, and so applying these concepts to carbohydrate counting (22,23,24) is compatible. After clients have experimented with hunger, fullness, satiety, meal mix, medication (oral and insulin), and resulting blood glucose levels, a preferred eating style emerges. Matching units of insulin to their preferred carbohydrate intake (measured in grams) can result in either tight or loose control, depending on clients' goals. This approach supports an internally-directed, nonrestrained style of eating while meeting clients' health goals.

HungerWork and Acute or Critical Care Clients

If a client's present weight or eating style seriously threatens health or exacerbates a medical condition, you and the client can discuss altering physical activity or eating style to go beyond the bounds of internal cues. A further consultation with the client and other health providers (physician, dietitian, therapist, exercise physiologist) may help weigh the costs and benefits of altering a satisfying eating style or activity preferences to offset health threats or problems.

If the alteration feels depriving or restricting, the client runs the risk of developing deprivation-driven eating or exercise resistance (See chapter on Joyful Movement for discussion of exercise resistance). Asking the client questions such as the ones below and exploring their views may elucidate potential issues. It is important that the client feels entitled to give genuine responses and is acknowledged for doing so:

> How do you feel about the proposed change in the way you eat? In the way you are physically active?
>
> Do you see a way to adapt to it slowly? How might slow change (if that is possible) affect your sense of deprivation or restriction?
>
> How do you feel about this disease (or condition) requiring you to sacrifice some pleasure and satisfaction in order to manage it?
>
> What do you understand might happen if you are unable or choose not to make these alterations?
>
> How might the decision not to make these changes affect your relationships (physicians, family members, friends)?
>
> How might you feel if you are able to maintain the new behaviors?
>
> How might you feel if you are not able to maintain the new behaviors?

SUMMARY OF HUNGERWORK WITH NUTRITION-SENSITIVE HEALTH PROBLEMS

Medical treatment that prescribes temporary restriction of food (as in gestational diabetes or liquid diets following gastric surgery) or compulsory exercise (as in re-adaptive or physical therapy following orthopedic surgery) poses some risk to clients in developing deprivation-driven eating or exercise resistance. Discussing this with clients before, during, and after the regimen may help offset some negative side-effects of restrained eating and compulsory exercise. However, they may not be avoidable.

Any suggestion to permanently restrict a person's freedom of choice in food and physical activity needs to be evaluated very carefully. Clients with nutrition-sensitive diseases experience deprivation due to their bodies' limited tolerance of certain foods and eating styles. Additionally, the individual may be deprived of some quality of health and/or longevity (1). Recommendations must be made on an individual basis rather than an idealized self-management regimen for an individual with that respective disease.

PUTTING IT ALL TOGETHER

An Eating Experience Reflecting the Three Facets of HungerWork

Imagine the potential freedom and deep satisfaction that comes from feeling entitled and designated to choose your own food **(internally-cued, nonrestrained eating)** that pleases your senses of taste, smell, sight, touch, sound **(joyful eating).** Connect these food choices with physical hunger **(identify internal cues),** temper the choice in a nonjudgmental way **(neutralize food)** with nutrition knowledge **(healthful eating).**

A client's decision-making process regarding when and what to eat may go something like this:

"Am I hungry? Yes."

"I'm really hungry, in fact I'm a 2."

"Do I choose to eat now at a 2, or is there an advantage to me if I wait?"

"Do I like the foods available to me now? Yes."

"Do I want hot or cold food? Sweet, salty, spicy, mild, soft, crunchy, chewy?"

"What are my senses asking for?"

"When did I have protein last?"

"How long do I need this meal to sustain me?"

"How do I want to feel at the end of this meal?"

"Am I familiar with how the available foods make me feel?"

"Is there an aroma I'm smelling that attracts me?"

"What do I want my food to look like?"

"What size portions would satisfy my hunger?"

"I'll choose..."

Over time, this procedure becomes natural. Until then, clients need us to model patience and acceptance of their decision-making processes, so in time they internalize self-caring attitudes. Remind your clients it is not natural for dieters to be physically-connected, trusting of their bodies' cues, unrestrained, and feel entitled to make their own food decisions. Constant support and positive feedback helps build self-confidence, furthers self-acceptance, leads to self-trust...and heals disconnection.

A Final Word

Eating well is one of life's greatest pleasures. Taste is the number one reason why people choose certain foods. A true, healthful eating style is a delicious balance of variety and moderation--healthy foods that look beautiful and taste great!

The new role of the health care provider is to find ways to expand choices rather than restrict choices while becoming pleasure promoters rather than pleasure restrictors. We need to blend the reasoning of the therapeutic world with the pleasures of the culinary world to promote a marriage of taste and health.

SELECTED RESOURCES

French Toast For Breakfast: Declaring Peace With Emotional Eating. MaryAnne Cohen. Carlsbad, CA: Gurze Books; 1995.

This book emphasizes the notion that people can be at peace with food. It not only explains the history of emotional eating, but also gives the reader practical guidelines in making changes which promote peaceful eating.

Games Diabetics Play...and How To Win Them. Joan Lyman. Santa Monica, CA: Wordsworth, projected release January 1997. (310)391-5175

Scripted by a psychotherapist with IDDM diabetes, these audio tapes (2) humorously, sensitively, and poignantly present the "games" individuals with diabetes find themselves playing and offer an empowering perspective shift in self-management. For example, "It Takes Two to Tango." This game requires having someone to blame, and a willingness to do it, "My partner won't let me eat correctly." How to be in charge of your food without declaring war.

Tailoring Your Tastes. Linda Omichinski and Heather Wiebe Hildebrand. Winnipeg, Manitoba: Tamos Books; 1995.

A wonderful cookbook which includes not only healthful recipes, but also a reasonable and gradual process of incorporating dietary changes into both the individual and family lifestyle. This book allows the cook to explore different tastes and preferences, while moving to a more health enhancing eating style.

Why Women Need Chocolate. Debra Waterhouse. New York, NY: Hyperion; 1995.
This book describes the role neurotransmitters, hormones, and other messengers play in cravings, appetite, and satisfaction. It emphasizes the importance of understanding these cravings and learning how to respond to them

REFERENCES

1. Bloom C, Gitter A, Gutwill S, Kogel L, Zaphiropoulos L. *Eating Problems: A Feminist Psychoanalytic Treatment Model.* New York, NY: Basic Books; 1994.
2. Satter E. *How to Get Your Kid to Eat...But Not Too Much.* Palo Alto, CA: Bull Publishing Company; 1987.
3. Position of the American Dietetic Association: Cost-effectiveness of medical nutrition therapy. *J Am Diet Assoc.* 1995; 95: 88-91.
4. Polivy J. Psychological consequences of food restriction. *J Am Diet Assoc.* 1996; 96:589-592.
5. Berg FM. *The Health Risks of Weight Loss, 3rd edition.* Hettinger, ND: Healthy Living Institute; 1995.
6. Blundell JE, Lawton CL, Hill AJ. Mechanisms of appetite control and their abnormalities in obese patients. *Horm-Res.* 1993; 39S: 72-76.
7. Kratina K. The core minimum daily food groups. In: *Disordered Eating Assessment and Treatment Tools.* Plantation, FL: Reflective Image, Inc.; 1993.
8. Robison JI, Hoerr SL, Petersmarck KA, Anderson JV. Redefining success in obesity prevention: The new paradigm. *J Am Diet Assoc.* 1995; 95: 422-423.
9. Stacey M. *Consumed: Why Americans Love, Hate, and Fear Food,* New York, NY: Touchstone; 1994.
10. Pomerleau J, Verdy M, Garrel DR; Nadeau MH. Effect of protein intake on glycemic control and renal function in type two (non-insulin-dependent) diabetes mellitus. *Diabetologia.* 1993; 36: 829.
11. King, NL. If Diets Don't Work, What Can Nutritional Professionals Do? Presentation. Am Diet Assoc. Annual Meeting and Exhibition. 1994. Orlando, FL.
12. Kissileff HR. Satiating efficiency and a strategy for conducting food loading experiments. *Neurosci Biobehav Rev.* 1984; 8: 129-135.
13. Blundell JE, Rogers PJ, Hill AJ. Evaluating the satiating power of foods: Implications for acceptance and consumption; in Solms J (ed): *Chemical Composition and Sensory Properties of Food and Their Influence on Nutrition.* London: Academic Press; 1987: 205-219.
14. Wikblad, Karin F. Montin, Kent R. Coping With a Chronic Disease. *The Diabetes Educator.* 1992; 18: 316-20.
15. Lyman JM, MA, MFCC. Personal communication. June 21, 1996. Pasadena, CA.
16. Hulshof T, De-Graaf C, Weststrate JA. The effects of preloads varying in physical states and fat content on satiety and energy intake. *Appetite.* 1993; 21: 273-86.
17. Allred JB. Too Much of a Good Thing: An overemphasis on eating low-fat foods may be contributing to the alarming increase in overweight among US adults. *J Am Diet Assoc.* 1995; 95 (4): 417-418.
18. The Diabetes Control and Complications Trial Research Group. The effect of intensive treatment of diabetes on the development and progression of long-term complications in insulin-dependent diabetes mellitus. *New Eng J of Med.* 1993; 329: 977-86.
19. Funnell MM, Anderson RM, Arnold MS, Barr PA, Donnelly M, Johnson PD, Taylor-Moon D, White NH. Empowerment: An idea whose time has come in diabetes education. *The Diabetes Educator.* 1991; 17: 37-41.
20. Wierenga ME, Beauchamp-Hewitt J. Facilitating Diabetes Self-Management. *The Diabetes Educator.* 1994; 20: 138-142.
21. The Diabetes Control and Complications Trial Research Group. Nutrition interventions for intensive therapy in the Diabetes Control and Complications Trial. *J Am Diet Assoc.* 1993; 768-772.
22. Tillotson LM, Shelton-Smith M. Locus of control, social support, and adherence to the diabetes regimen. *The Diabetes Educator.* 1996; 22: 133-139.
23. Walker EA. A response on patient empowerment and the medical model. *Diabetes Spectrum.* 1995; 8: 188.
24. Gregory R, Davis D. Use of carbohydrate counting for meal planning Type I diabetes. *The Diabetes Educator.* 1994; 20: 406-409.
25. Daly A, Barry B, Gillespie S, Kulkarni K, Richardson M. *Carbohydrate Counting: Using carbohydrate/insulin ratios.* American Dietetic Association/American Diabetes Association, 1995.
26. Daly A. Carbohydrate Counting: New Teaching Resources. *Practical Diabetology.* 1996; 15: 19-23

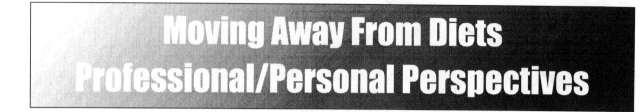

Moving Away From Diets
Professional/Personal Perspectives

Linda O., Registered Dietitian, Manitoba, Canada

Some people say that only frustrated professionals want this approach, that clients don't want it.
People often have to hear the message several times before they "buy into" taking a program of this kind since the message is new and foreign to them.

I remember one individual calling me up after being on the radio ready to break the diet cycle and in speaking with her, she asked me if I was on a particular TV show two years ago. She went on to indicate that she was only listening with one ear at that time and she wasn't quite ready yet. The good news is that there is a momentum building and more and more people are beginning to speak out and welcome an approach which no longer makes them feel like they failed. Just as it takes health professionals a process to move from the continuum of using the diet medical model to the nondiet empowerment model, it takes individuals time to give up dieting, something that has been comfortable and familiar to them for a good part of their lives.

What personal/professional experiences led you to move to a nondieting paradigm?
The recognition that I was doing more harm than good by continuing to use the diet approach that I had learned in my training as a dietitian. My experience has been that it is often difficult for health professionals to give up the familiar diet approach that they have been trained to deliver as this is within their comfort zone.

It's scary to give up the individualized diet model as then there is a learning curve that presents itself and it feels like you are starting over again. Health professionals are then up against learning new skills and a new approach and sometimes it's just easier to keep on going with what you know than to take on this new challenge. To make this process easier, it's important for these health professionals to realize that this transition takes time and to take smaller steps in gradually introducing some nondiet concepts into one's counseling and see how it feels. As one begins to notice that their clients experience a sense of freedom and their counseling becomes more effective and satisfying, they will choose to learn more about the approach and eventually deliver programs that are totally nondiet. It took me several years of reading, researching, networking, attending conferences and experimenting before I completely adopted a nondiet approach. Acknowledge the little steps first and in time, this new way of looking at food and life will become internalized skills that transfer into every part of your life.

Leslie M., Administrator, Tujunga, CA

Has using a nondiet approach changed your life? In what ways?
Yes. I'm not obsessing about food! It's a releasing, freeing feeling when I'm not obsessing about food. When am I going to eat again? What am I going to eat? Can I last that long? Can I be that far away from food? Will I be okay? Can I go somewhere and not know when I'll be able to eat again?

What goals do you have for the future in terms of these issues?
Reach my natural weight. Not binge. Eat when hungry and stop when full.

7
Joyful Movement

> What happened?
> One day you're strolling
> around in the buff and
> looking the world straight
> in the eye without
> so much as a blush.
> Then wallop!
> Puberty. Boys.
> Magazine images.
> Suddenly the mirror is no
> longer your friend.
> So who defined your
> template of beauty?
> Who said you weren't OK?
> Get real.
> Make your body the best
> it can be for one person.
> Yourself.
> *Just do it.*
>
> *Nike. Used with permission.*

HUNGER FOR MOVEMENT

People are born with a "hunger for movement." As infants and children we enjoy our bodies and experience exquisite joy when we move, whether we fall or not. We delight in squirming, exploring, grasping, throwing and tumbling. As children we run, hide, jump, skip, invent games, throw balls and squirm when sitting still. At this time in our lives, we are not self-conscious about the way we look or whether we are doing it right. We move and play because it feels good and it is fun.

Some people stay involved in sports learned in childhood, or they pick up new fitness activities as an adult. They keep a passion for activity that fuels their desire to move, explore and play.

Others of us however, dramatically shift the relationship between our bodies and movement. Through the teenage years and into adulthood we quit moving; quit enjoying our bodies. Maybe we are told "it isn't lady-like," or we get busy with school or a job. Our muscles lose strength and our bodies lose endurance. When we play an occasional volleyball game, throw a Frisbee or run after a bus, we feel it. We become winded and uncomfortable. The next day our bodies might feel sore. We say "our bodies rebelled," and we back further away from movement.

COUNSELING QUANDRY

As a counselor, if you have never lost the hunger for movement (even though you may have quit exercising for extended periods of time), it may be hard to understand a client without that spark. You may recommend that clients walk 3 times a week for 20 minutes. You may conduct a fitness assessment followed by a personalized exercise prescription or refer your client for this workup. Logically, it seems that if clients know *what* exercises to do, how *much* to do and understand *why it is needed,* they will be motivated and will follow through.

> ***Joyless exercise repeated as a daily ritual dampens the spirit*** *(1).*

Considering that less than 20% of adults in the U.S. exercise regularly, this knowledge or awareness does not seem to be enough. Some clients will follow the guidelines and find they enjoy exercise and continue. For the majority, however, the spark never ignites. They do not reconnect with their body and they do not find joy in movement. They may follow their exercise prescription for awhile, but experience it as joyless activity, drudgery, a way to reach some distant, possibly unachieveable goal, and they soon quit.

We may assume the ones who quit are too lazy, not committed enough, or did not prioritized their life effectively. In fact, they may have no spark. It's not fun. They find no joy in moving their bodies; it is just something they have to do. Without that joy in movement, they will find something else to do that is more fun. If they are exercising for weight loss, and they do not see the numbers on the scale dropping, they will find a more rewarding way to spend their time.

WHY WOULDN'T SOMEONE WANT TO MOVE?

Because of the hype, many people feel discouraged; they can't achieve the ideal prescription of vigorous exercise sessions, and the sleek look of the sinewy models glowing out of magazines covers some how evades them. So they do nothing (1).

It is important to be nonjudgmental about a client's sedentary lifestyle. It is also important to understand there are a myriad of reasons a client is not moving. Asking open-ended questions while exploring a client's relationship with activity can assist in understanding the reasons for their sedentary lifestyle.

The following are just some of the reasons people quit moving. Consider the following situations in an effort to understand avoidance of movement. Consider how each may impact an individual.

- As a child, they were picked last by teams and felt rejected. They were picked on or made fun of while performing an activity, or told they were not coordinated. Eventually they *believed* they were not good enough and "I'm a clutz" became their *mantra.*
- Growing up, they felt extreme pressure to perform from their parents, physical education teachers or coaches. Or, they had perfectionistic tendancies and when they could not reach their own or others' high standards, they moved away from physical activity believing, "I can't do it right, so I won't do it."
- They were repeatedly pushed into exercise; maybe someone wanted them to "have fun" or wanted to help them lose weight. Avoiding activity may be, albeit subconsciously, a way of rebelling against those who pushed them, against the subtle message, "You are not OK as you are."
- They felt pain and rejection when someone berated their bodies, and on some level, decided to move their bodies as little as possible to attract the least amount of attention possible.
- They were injured and have a fear of exercise, especially if the injury occurred during an activity they felt tentative about.
- They exercised only when dieting, when their energy was low. The activity was started with lethargy and minimal enthusiasm.
- They exercise only when they diet to lose weight. When they quit dieting, they also quit exercising. Exercise becomes a necessary evil, one which they return to with the next diet.

- They start exercise programs with an all or nothing attitude, believing they must push to the max to get benefit. Or they may believe if they miss a day of their routine they have blown it. They may not realize the minimal amounts of activity needed to improve health. They end up quitting because they think they are not doing any good anyway.
- They attempt an exercise program, but do not understand how to do the exercises (it takes time to be able to exercise correctly, especially if one has been sedentary). They feel intimidated by equipment or the fancy moves in aerobics classes.

I've been trying to add more activity into my life too. I use a student fitness center at the University where I am a grad student and all of the other people there are at least 15 years younger than me. I realized that being around that age group (18-22) is too hard for me. Some of them are very critical and I even caught two young "jocks" whispering and laughing at me... and for those of you who wonder how I know they were addressing me... you just KNOW (3).

- They try to make time for exercise but feel overwhelmed by the demands of life. Exercise at that time becomes an impossibility in their mind, "I'll start exercising when the kids are in school."
- They feel rejection from a friend, family or society, believing the rejection is due to the size/shape of their bodies. They then use exercise to change their body. They become disappointed in themselves as well as with exercise when they don't become that ideal shape.
- They use exercise as an external measure of self-worth. In our culture, exercise is revered as something that supposedly reflects on an individual's inner character, a testimony to their strength and inner worth (4). Rebellion is common when exercise is used this way.
- They punish themselves with exercise when they perceive they eat too much, or don't lose enough weight. Punishment is always remembered as negative. Exercise then, has negative connotations.

One client followed a 1200 calorie meal plan. She added the calories she consumed each day and noted any overage. Then she added up any calories over 1200 for the week and calculated how many hours she would need to bicycle to burn off the calories. Every Sunday, she got up at 6:30 to bicycle away excess calories. She felt very positive about this burning of calories, stating she was doing something good for herself. Unfortunately, she saw exercise only as a means of burning calories and was not enjoying the early morning ride. She was able to continue this for only 5 weeks, when she quit exercising altogether.

- They experienced sexual abuse. Moving the body can bring up body memories of the abuse. Exercise can trigger flashbacks of repressed abuse. It can be restimulating due to the movement of the body, being warm or sweating, or simply because the abuse took place in the body and in some way, the trauma is stored there (4). Exercising is often curtailed after abuse begins, at puberty or at some point when an individual experiences being sexually objectified. See Chapter 8 for an example of this. It is important to remember that not all large people were sexually abused. Also, the abuse need not be overt.

Occasionally, individuals are able to recreate their body in the shape they desire. Usually these individuals began with some decent genes (Jane Fonda), they added a trainer who worked them out for 5 ½ hours a day (Linda Hamilton), they hired a "nutritionist" to plan their menus (Cher), they hired a chef to cook their food (Oprah Winfrey), they underwent corrective surgery (Demi Moore), they use their sculpted bodies as a source of income (Cory Everson), and maybe they starved (Kate Moss?). Oh yeah, and maybe in the meanwhile they were preparing for a movie in which they would gross 10 million dollars. Most likely these individuals will be able to make and remake their bodies at their whim...for a while. Meanwhile, the rest of us (the other 99.9% of the world population) don't have the time, money, incentives or genes to accomplish this feat. Those that decide to try anyway are often disappointed in themselves as well as with exercise when they don't become their concept of an ideal shape. They don't realize the odds were against them from the beginning.

> *As a teenager I was still serious about dance. My teachers liked that. But I was also slinking around, trying to hide the parts of my body that were too big. I was always the largest one in class. No one ever sat me down and said, "You can't be a dancer, you're too big." But I got that message loud and clear every day. I never progressed to the advanced class. When we had demonstrations, I was never given good parts, I was placed in the back, behind everyone else.*
>
> *I spent years trying to figure out why my teachers were hard on me. I think they saw potential in me but felt thwarted because I had the "wrong" body type. Sometimes they were downright cruel. I was rarely praised for what I did well, but I was criticized for not having my leg high enough or not bending back far enough. No one ever thought to acknowledge that my body made it harder for me. In class, I saw praise go to the students who didn't work half as hard as I did, simply because they were thin and long and lithe. And I was confused, because although I was willing to give up all my free time outside of school to sweat in a dance class, I was considered lazy, unmotivated, and undisciplined. Even though I often went home in tears, I never stopped going to class. I loved to dance. It allowed me to express myself with my body-through the movement, the music, the discipline, and hard work* (2).

- Presenting an exercise prescription may motivate some resistent individuals initially, but unless the individual can connect with the exercise and finds some enjoyment, the prescription will probably be useless.

FINDING JOY IN ACTIVITY

> *Moving your body means returning to the joy of childhood play. It means forgetting all the rules and shoulds about exercise, and changing the concept from grueling work-out to zestful play-time. Moving your body is one of the best ways to keep physical hunger signals on cue and to naturally lift sagging spirits* (5).

Zestful playtime?? What does it mean to be playful? We recognize it when we see it. We remember playfulness instinctively. Playfulness is a letting go, a freedom from self-consciousness, from the shoulds and have-to's, and an awakening of the spirit that lives in each of us (1).

Some may find it odd to talk about play in the same context as exercise. This misconception is one of the travesties of the fitness movement (1). To be fit, we are advised to follow a formula, maybe an expert-created exercise routine. This isn't wrong, it is just not the whole picture. There are other choices (1).

We suggest that a key to rediscovering pleasure in movement is to quit compulsory exercise, throw out the rules and shoulds, and start moving for fun. This does not mean throwing out structured exercise, unless it is not enjoyable. If your clients are doing structured exercise, make sure they are thoroughly enjoying it!!

BUT WHAT ABOUT HEALTH?

> *There are people who will argue to the death that fat people cannot be healthy and fit, that the terms fat and fit are mutually exclusive. While experts will continue to disagree, even contradict one another on the actual health risks of fat, you need not wait for their consensus to become more fit and healthy regardless of your weight* (6).

As mentioned earlier, health is an important consideration in the nondiet approach. We hope to challenge the belief many professionals have that adopting a nondiet approach means giving clients permission to sit in front of the TV eating Twinkies for the rest of their, albeit short, lives.

Think in terms of giving permission. In traditional health care, the professional is in charge, dictating the behaviors necessary for the client. The professional is the change agent, while the client becomes the passive recipient of the advice. As noted in Chapter 1, this is how most of us were taught to work with clients. For some clients, this is fine; they make the changes. For others, change does not occur. In fact, many people rebel when given advise...including a high percentage of us who give the advice. We suggest moving from advice-giving to guiding our clients. Rather than prescribing, advising, allowing or disallowing behaviors as we were taught to do, we need to guide our clients in the exploration of movement, exercise and the adoption of healthy lifestyles. Chapter 8 discusses this further.

Yes, exercise is extremely important to health, but exercise is a loaded term in our culture. We need to approach this issue gently.

> *I REALLY and truly believe that exercise is as large and loaded an issue as food--as big, as unwieldy, as pervasive, as skewed as food--due to the way it's presented, how it's (ab)used for weight loss, how we've experienced it; the fact that it is a vital part of the current beauty ideal... And for this reason, I do think we need to do with exercise exactly what we're doing with food: remove all rules, all pressures and goals, and try very hard to listen to what our bodies are saying at the moment. Just at the moment, not in any kind of long-range way. I also think that the fact that exercise is as big an issue as food means it requires just as much work to debunk (not the right word, but I can't think of anything else right now)* (3).

INVENTION OF EXERCISE.....the concentrated cure for not being active all day

The very notion of exercise guidelines was preposterous a few generations ago, when most people got all the activity they needed doing what had to be done: washing the clothes in a tub, walking miles to school, plowing and harvesting by hand, and so on.

Then came cars and electric motors, washing machines and TV remote controls, resulting in sedentary lifestyles. Studies show that a sedentary lifestyle leads to poor health. If we can no longer get enough activity in our daily lives, we have to invent a way to get it if we want to be healthy. So exercise was invented. In the 1970's, scientists first collaborated to determine how much exercise was necessary for good health.

Notions about fitness have changed a great deal since that time. In 1975, experts recommended we work out hard enough to reach at least 60 percent of VO_2 max (which would require running, high-impact aerobics, bicycling racing, etc). By 1984, the level of intensity fell to 50 percent. More recent guidelines suggest we workout at 40 percent VO_2 max (a fast paced walk) (7).

It turns out that it takes relatively little exercise to improve health for most individuals. Several studies have found that exercisers who don't drop a pound still live longer and healthier lives (8,9,10). It is not even because they lowered their cholesterol or blood pressure, studies show that even when those indices remain the same, moderate exercisers get protection against heart disease and stroke.

Interestingly, Carrier, Steinhardt and Bowman (11) found that individuals who were supported in moving away from dieting not only exhibited an increase in self-esteem and self-acceptance, they also had increased levels of physical activity at a 3 year follow-up.

While previous guidelines required a minimum of 30 minutes of serious exercise five days a week with no playing around (for example, 3 days of running, bicycling, aerobics, swimming plus 2 days of calisthenics), the new guidelines have lightened up. "Exercise Lite," the latest exercise recommendations issued jointly by the U.S. Centers for Disease Control and Prevention and the American College of Sports Medicine (7) still recommends 30 minutes of activity at least 5 times a week; however, play now counts! Anything from throwing a Frisbee to roughhousing with the kids can be considered physical activity, and it does not all have to be completed at the same time. Scientific research shows that health benefits are most impacted by the total quantity of physical activity on a given day rather than the type, duration and intensity of the activity (7).

Some sedentary people believe that if they can't do it right, there is no point doing it at all. With these new guidelines, improved health and fitness are closer than previously thought. As our clients realize that a little movement adds up to big benefits, especially in the beginning, they may be more willing to engage in physical activity.

The Exercise/Diet Combo

It is a popular notion that we need to exercise and diet to be healthy. However, most people do not know about the negative ramifications of combining exercise with restrained eating to manage body shape. A 1990 study revealed there may be a direct relationship between regular participation in a fitness program and excessive concern with the body, weight and dieting (12). A subsequent study found that those who exercise with high frequency had a significantly more negative view of their bodies than did moderate and non-exercisers (13). A negative perception of one's body is known to fuel dieting behavior as well as the development of eating disorders. In fact, it has been suggested that the pressure to combine diet and exercise to reduce body weight is a precipitant to the development of eating disorders (14). These researchers propose that, of those that develop anorexia, 75% have done so because they have combined intense dieting with exercise.

It has also been found that, for some individuals, the combination of structured exercise and dietary restraint may cause both activities to become driven (15). These behaviors may be perpetuated by physiological changes which make them resistant to intervention. These individuals may become reclusive, anxious, and depressed. High-achieving, productive men and women are prone to develop these difficulties (15).

FYI...WHAT THE AMERICAN COLLEGE OF SPORTS MEDICINE RECOMMENDS

For Cardio-Respiratory Fitness

Improvement in cardiorespiratory function depends upon the intensity, duration, and frequency of the training program. The American College of Sports Medicine recommends the following for the enhancement of health and cardiorespiratory fitness (16):

(1) Mode of activity: Any activity that uses large muscle groups that can be maintained for a prolonged period and is rhythmic and aerobic in nature, e.g. running, jogging, walking, hiking, swimming, skating, bicycling, rowing, cross-country skiing, rope skipping or various endurance games.

(2) Intensity of exercise: Physical activities corresponding to 40 to 85 percent VO2 max or 55 to 90 percent of maximal heart rate. It should be noted that exercise of low-end intensity may provide important health benefits and may result in increased fitness in some persons (e.g. those who were previously sedentary and low fit).

(3) Duration of exercise: 30 to 60 minutes of continuous or discontinuous aerobic activity

(4) Frequency of exercise: Three to five days per week.

(5) Rate of progression: In most cases the conditioning effect allows individuals to increase the total work done per session. In continuous exercise this occurs by an increase in intensity, duration or by some combination of the two. The most significant conditioning effects may be observed during the first 6 to 8 weeks of the exercise program. The exercise prescription may be adjusted as these conditioning effects occur with the adjustment depending on participant characteristics, the exercise test results and/or exercise performance during exercise sessions.

For Strength and Endurance

Muscular strength and endurance are developed by the overload principle. The American College of Sports Medicine (16) recommends strength training, two times a week, completing 8 to 10 exercises working the major muscle groups, a minimum of one set of 8 to 12 repetitions. Muscular strength is best developed through the use of heavy weights with few repetitions and muscular endurance is best developed by using lighter weights with a greater number of repetitions. Doing more than the recommended does not dramatically increase fitness. One study compared individuals who trained two days a week to those who trained 3 days a week, and found an increase in strength of 20% and 28% respectively after 18 weeks (17). In other words, 75% of what could be attained exercising three days a week was attained exercising two days a week.

HOW IS EXERCISE DIFFERENT FOR LARGE BODIES?

Remember that fatness does not preclude fitness. Thin people aren't always fit, nor heavy people necessarily unfit. The great dancer Isadora Duncan was a "big woman" and 200 pound Virgina Zucci, of the Russian Ballet, was famous for her pirouettes. Lynne Cox, who swam the English Channel and broke the women's record by three hours, the men's record by one hour, is 5'6" and 180# (and 33% body fat). The winner of the 1994 Nike Fitness Leader of the Year Award was a large women named De Dast-Hakala who teaches step aerobics and champions the cause of large women. Heavy women need to move as much as anyone else (18).

It is interesting to note that while fat people are more likely to get certain kinds of heart disease than thin people (especially chest pains from angina), these kinds of heart disease are also common in people who are inactive, regardless of their weight. This could mean that the reason more fat people have these kinds of heart disease is that more fat people are inactive. If so, there is no reason to believe that an active fat person is a better candidate for a coronary than an equally active thin person (19).

One study found that large women engaged in regular exercise who showed no weight loss (in fact there was an average of 2 pound gain), reduced their blood pressures (10). E*xercise promotes health even in those who remain much heavier than doctors' weight charts suggest is healthy.*

Activity For The Ample-Bodied

When discussing physical activity with the ample-bodied, we need to remember that big bodies are different and movements need to be designed with that difference in mind. Exercises should be low-impact, since added weight puts extra stress on joints, magnifying the danger of strains from improper exercise routines. The larger an individual is, the more demanding each movement. A larger person's body has to work harder than an average person's body doing the same work. It also consumes more oxygen for each movement.

Unfortunately, many people have been told by health providers that being heavy "puts a strain on your heart." In fact, this is often cited as one of the evils of being overweight. Actually, added weight is the reason why it is easier for a fat person to get aerobic exercise. A heavy person who walks can get the same intensity of workout as a thin person who runs. As with anyone, more exertion is needed to get the heart rate up as fitness level increases. However, keep in mind that a heavy individual may never have to do more than walk to receive significant health benefits.

While there are formulas used to determine the target heart rate at which an individual should be exercising for maximal benefit, caution is advised when using them. Some clients may enjoy the scientific aspect of monitoring exercise heart rate and watching resting heart rate decrease over time while learning about its impact on health. For others, this would be too reminiscent of the ineffective formulas given to them for weight loss. The 'talk test' in which one exercises just hard enough to be able to carry on a conversation while moving may be all that is necessary.

Heavy people do face some special difficulties when exercising. Fat tissue acts as insulation, trapping the heat generated by exercise inside the body. During a workout, very large people can become feverish and feel ill. This is why it's especially important for big people to wear absorbent clothing that allows air to circulate over the skin and to workout in a cool, well-ventilated environment. Also, fat deposits in the chest area make deep breaths more difficult, so the diaphragm must do more work and become stronger. To avoid the extra effort of taking deep breaths, many heavy people tend to take rapid, shallow breaths. They become uncomfortable when first starting to exercise because they've forgotten how to breathe deeply. With regular exercise, fat people strengthen their diaphragms and learn to breathe more deeply, even when not exercising (19).

Large individuals also need to thoroughly warm-up their lower legs, ankles and feet before they begin moving. Warming up while sitting in chairs puts less stress on the lower back. The surface upon which an individual exercises has a great deal to do with how their body will feel. This is an especially important consideration for a large person. Unfortunately, many are quick to blame this on weight and not explore other areas. Weight is a factor, however, we cannot stop there. If unexplained aches and pains are getting in the way of activity, ask your client to try different surfaces. Cement or blacktop have

> Remember, a large person can be moving substantially slower than a small person while incurring the same work load. Years ago I worked at a small eating disorders unit housed in an acute care hospital. The nature of the facility made it difficult to exercise outdoors, and since there was no exercise equipment, patients walked on the unit. While the large patients appeared to be ambling, they were doing as much work as the thinner patients. I was horrified to hear the staff making fun of the larger patients. Unfortunately, this typifies the ignorance of many health care practitioners. Karin Kratina

no "give," which results in the body absorbing the impact of each step. Recommend dirt trails, grassy meadows or trails with pine needles, sand closest to the water at a beach, and so on.

There are movements which large individuals simply may *not* be able to do, such as:

- lifting the knee up;
- reaching behind themselves and interlace hands;
- putting elbows together in front of bust;
- crossing legs in front of each other to move sideways;
- quick changes in direction and hasty pivots;
- some stretching exercises while standing;
- certain types of weight lifting.

Explore this with your client. It may be such a common occurrence for them that they would not think to discuss it, or they may be embarrassed. In any case, these issues can interfere with regular exercise and discussion of these issues may benefit the client.

> *Next I tried an Afro-Caribbean dance class, which had great music and great dance steps.*
> *The instructor was somewhat supportive, but I couldn't keep up with the rigorous warm-up*
> *for most of the dance moves, which hurt my back. I retreated back into a life with no dance*
> *and no movement, but my longing remained (2).*

Clothing

Help your client find clothes that are comfortable, make them feel good about themselves and meet the needs of whatever activity they are doing. Clothes should allow for freedom of movement, be absorbent and breathable. Lycra and cotton-lycra blends tights can help reduce irritation when legs rub together. They can be worn under shorts or skirts. *Great Shapes* (6) recommends putting petroleum gel on the inner thighs to reduce chafing when wearing shorts. Sweat pants also work. A bra that fits with wide straps and is designed for sports will add to comfort. Shoes that fit with extra toe space designed for activity are also important. Velcro closures make shoes easier to put on and take off.

I KNOW WHAT TO DO, I JUST DON'T DO IT...EXERCISE RESISTANCE

We can explain to our clients why they need activity, how much better they will feel with activity, and so on, but when a client has resistance to physical activity, these are mute points. Occasionally clients may not understand or accept the necessity of moving, or of the possibility of enjoying it. Usually this is the result of significant exercise resistance brought on by situations similar to those mentioned at the beginning of the chapter. One strategy used to solve this dilemma is to ask the client to commit to getting no activity for a specified, or even unspecified period of time. Any educating is then undertaken gently while underlying issues are explored. It is helpful to explore the impact of lack of movement on their life while they are not exercising. Use Figure 7-A to help clients identify where they are on the Movement Continuum.

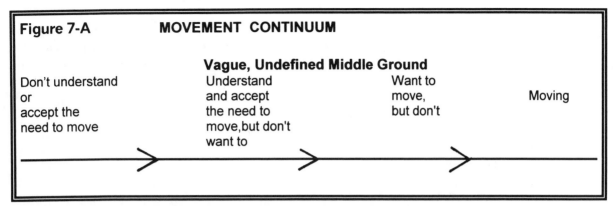

Figure 7-A **MOVEMENT CONTINUUM**

Vague, Undefined Middle Ground

| Don't understand or accept the need to move | Understand and accept the need to move,but don't want to | Want to move, but don't | Moving |

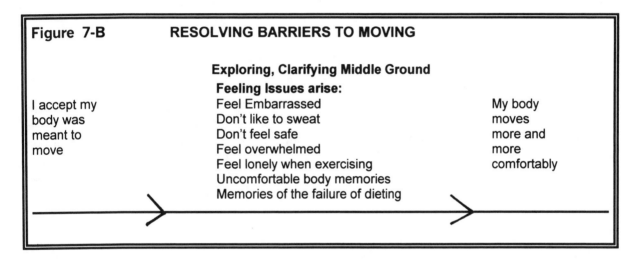

Figure 7-B **RESOLVING BARRIERS TO MOVING**

Exploring, Clarifying Middle Ground
Feeling Issues arise:

| I accept my body was meant to move | Feel Embarrassed
Don't like to sweat
Don't feel safe
Feel overwhelmed
Feel lonely when exercising
Uncomfortable body memories
Memories of the failure of dieting | My body moves more and more comfortably |

As the following chart, Figure 7-B, shows, clients may understand the need to move but do not want to, or more confusing, they may want to but do not. Many times these clients are not able to figure out why they cannot get there. They are stuck somewhere between the knowing and the doing.

The health professional will need to access the feelings in the middle ground. The fears and disappointments, the rules and formulas, the pain and shame will need to be explored if the client is to enjoy joyful movement. A skilled health professional can successfully process many of these issues. However, knowledge of the limits of one's scope of practice is critical. For instance, if a client is experiencing uncomfortable body memories, they will need to be referred to a psychotherapist. Following is a typical case study showing a nutrition therapist moving a client through exercise resistance.

Beth is a 52 year old homemaker, who has been in psychotherapy and nutrition therapy for four years. She is 5'6" and weighs 260#. Having been a dieter for many years, Beth is dealing with deprivation-driven and emotional eating. Through neutralizing food, lifting food restrictions and experimenting with food, she stopped binge eating. Occasionally, Beth will get on food jags that last a week or two, but her weight remains stable, within 4 pounds over the last 3 years.

Beth is aware of her body's changes due to her weight and lack of physical activity. She is losing her mobility. She has difficulty getting in and out of her car and dressing in the morning. Running errands leaves her exhausted. Initially she believed the problem was her excess weight. While it is true that being large can limit mobility and cause tiredness, every diet Beth went on left her larger. The nutrition therapist understood weight loss is a moot point at best and continually redirected Beth to look at the issue of fitness. Beth occasionally thinks she "should" be exercising, but puts the notion out of her mind immediately. She admits she is a slow learner.

Recently, she shared much of what she doesn't like about exercise, especially the "shoulds" with her nutrition therapist. Processing these thoughts and feelings, it became apparent that for her, the very idea of obligation to exercise is enough reason to resist.

As they explored various kinds of movement, Beth said she likes the way water feels, "it's gentle, smooth, supportive." She was encouraged to spend time near as many bodies of water (including ponds, and bird baths) as often as possible.

As a form of therapy, Beth agreed to create and write down a conversation with the water. What would she say? If water could talk, what would she want to know about water as it relates to her? Beth started with asking the water if it would be gentle, smooth, and supportive of her if she got in it. She asked her body if it would find this comforting.

Beth decided to go to the YMCA to watch the swimmers and water aerobic exercise classes. (A spark of interest in movement!) Both groups of exercisers spoke to her and by the time she got home, she was searching for catalogues for exercise equipment for large size women. (Another spark of interest!) She found one, and proceeded to order two bathing suits. (Another spark!) She kept the bathing suits in her dresser. Six months later, she got up one morning and decided it was the day to try the class. She did, and found she thoroughly enjoyed it. That was 9 months ago and she is still "in the water." She found that her mobility has increased dramatically as has her energy levels. Her weight never changed.

To help clients overcome exercise resistance, first help them reconnect with the fun of moving their bodies. After their physicians assess and approve moderate exercise, do not confuse the issue and overwhelm clients with checking heart rates. Forget about how many minutes someone *should* exercise, forget about how many times a week, and forget about having the RIGHT form, although always reinforce safety. Let's help our clients get back into the experience first, help them learn to have fun, to play, to move. Let's help them get more comfortable moving their bodies...paying attention to their bodies request for movement. Let's help empower them to make the changes.

So many things surrounding exercise scare me. Before seeing my counselor, going to the gym would be lumped in with the idea that I needed some sort of life change (even then I don't think I recognized that the impetus was often just that I needed to move!!). And after an experience like today, I'd always say, "now, that was good, but to be <u>really</u> good, I should do this x times a week building up to this many minutes (miles, whatever), blah, blah, blah." I'm terrified of that conversation that happens with myself and all the stress that goes along with it. I know that it's the same as a diet even if I'm not thinking weight loss (3).

SIMPLE, FUN MOVEMENT
Fitness should be pleasurable and, unfortunately, popular health advice often ignores less intense, more enjoyable forms of physical activity (20).

Help clients think of pleasurable activities that can be done in the course of the day, as part of life, and preferably without structure. For example, gardening, hoeing, digging, pulling weeds, and pushing a lawn mower can increase heart rates by 20 to 25%; for a sedentary person, this may be enough of a boost to improve health (20). An occasional swim, bouncing up and down in a swimming pool, a wild dance, batting a tennis ball back and forth with a friend, hitting a racket ball against a backboard, bowling, playing catch or Frisbee with a friend all can increase one's heart rate and may be health enhancing. Walk the dog. Take an extra spin around the mall when shopping. Carry all the groceries from the car rather than ask for help. Take a dance class. Play with the children or get down on all fours and chase the dog around. Rake leaves, shovel snow, push a lawn mower. Make love. Gardening gets you outside and, instead of running nowhere, you end up growing something new, something alive (20). Walk with a goal that has nothing to do with exercise. For instance, pick flowers along the way and plan to come home with a little bouquet of flowers for your dining room table. Plan some new landscaping by looking for ideas along the way. Be the judge of a contest to pick the house in the neighborhood with the best grass, cleanest windows or prettiest walkway (18).

Great Shapes, a fitness book for large women, suggests that fitness activities be (6):

1. familiar,
2. accessible to most people,
3. pleasurable,
4. challenging in such a way that an individual can push or back off depending on their needs,
5. very low risk.

A WORD ABOUT HARASSMENT

The pleasures, benefits, challenges, and full-out exuberant fun of dance, sport, and movement are the birthrights of all people, not just the already athletic and fit. But larger women have been treated shabbily by the exercise establishment. Regardless of any polite veneer, the fat-hating attitudes of most instructors would make even the most stalwart believer in self-esteem cringe under their judgment. And it is very difficult to separate their hatred of the substance fat from their feelings toward you, a fat person (6).

As stated earlier, it is probably the existence of prejudice and discrimination toward fat people that most severely undermines their health and well-being. They also keep many large individuals from becoming more physically active, and more healthy. We need to understand and help our clients deal with the victimization that occurs with these attitudes. We must revisit our own opinions and attitudes, and move on to help change those of our peers, other professionals and society at large.

Large women have begun to form their own groups where they can perform activities without having to risk rude comments, stares or being ostracized by others. There are groups that enjoy swimming, biking, canoeing, cross country ski trips, dance, aerobics, belly dance, hikes, and so on.

Now I teach the [large woman's dance class]. I love putting on an outrageous spandex leotard and tights and leading the class. I love being able to tell large women, "It's okay to be yourself here. You look great!" The atmosphere we have created is supportive and noncompetitive. We don't say, "Get your leg up higher," and "Move faster," as they do in other aerobic classes. Wherever your leg is, is fine. We focus on proper alignment to avoid injury and on having fun. It gives me a thrill to see a class of beautiful, large women dancing their hearts out (2).

Discrimination and Fear of Humiliation

Unfortunately, few people who have not "been there" can ever fully realize what it is like to live in a fat phobic culture. The issues of prejudice and discrimination come up much too frequently when large individuals attempt to increase their activity. As discussed earlier, it is difficult to imagine the level at which large people are left out in our society. This rejection is overwhelming even when we look at one small area of life...fitness and exercise opportunities. Consider a large person's attempt to fit in at the gym:

- They are often stared at and talked about.
- Jokes are made at their expense, often loud enough for them to hear.
- The seats on the stationary bikes are too small and uncomfortable.
- The stationary bikes, and other aerobic equipment are too close together to maneuver between comfortably.
- Weight machines do not fit so they cannot be used comfortably, or at all.
- Getting up from the floor and low equipment is extremely difficult.

- Aerobics classes are usually designed for the individual who can and wants to move intensely. Even when told to "modify the movements, go at your own pace," many do not know how to do this. Even if they did, once again they do not fit in.

> Following is an example of one client's experience:
> *After working with a nutrition therapist for 8 months, Jerri, a 28 year old woman who was 5'7" and weighed 217#, finally got up the nerve to visit a gym where she had been a member for four months. In the locker room as she was putting her things in a locker, stowing the courage to workout, a woman said to her (this is a direct quote), "You're disgusting. Why don't you do something about yourself."*
> Needless to say she didn't go back.

Why is it large people are shamed while trying to do what everyone thinks they should be doing?

FIT AND FAT: AN IDEA WHOSE TIME HAS COME (6)

> *I finished the 7.6 mile course in one hour forty-five minutes. There are those who say "real" runners go much faster than that, but what did I care? I wasn't even supposed to be able to run. I was labeled* obese *by medical types, and three months after I'd started running I read in a fitness book that people more than thirty pounds "overweight" shouldn't run, that they should lose weight before running. Fortunately I read that after I'd discovered the challenge, exuberance, and rewards of running, or I might never have had the Bay to Breakers [run] to celebrate. I was fat but I was fit, and no one could take that away from me (6).*

Now is the time to question our "truths" we were taught about being fit and fat. Being thin does not guarantee health or fitness. There are 150# men and 110# women who cannot walk a mile in 12 minutes or swim one lap of a pool. Being fat doesn't mean that muscles, lungs, fuel systems and other elements of the fitness formula cannot be trained to work efficiently. There are 200# women who can swim longer and faster than men; clinically obese men who can climb a flight of stairs without getting winded, and 250# women who can dance for hours and do splits. In other words, fat people can be fit.

Given what large women have had to put up with, we need to respect their right *not* to exercise. "Remember that exercise is not a duty of fat people. They have no more obligation to exercise than anyone else. We need to *invite* our clients to become more active. We believe that large women can and do enjoy exercise but only when we are treated, and treat ourselves, with respect. Physical activity is a way to nourish our bodies, not reduce them; a way to enrich our lives, not punish ourselves (6)."

COUNSELING STRATEGIES: FACILITATING THE CHANGE

> *When we accept ourselves as we are today and gradually proceed to make the changes we want for ourselves, we have more power to recreate our lives. When we are self-accepting, we love ourselves for not being perfect already. The burden of self-rejection makes it very hard to change our lives.* Yogi Desai (1)

Counseling needs to focus on a clients' past relationship with exercise and their current relationship with their bodies, while exploring options to find and reconnect with the joy of movement. It may not be necessary to discover the root of exercise resistance; however, understanding the clients past experiences will assist in guiding them towards joyful movement. Francie White, MS, RD, recommends that health care providers (21):

1. Initially explore and validate exercise resistance as a pattern of dropping exercises for reasons that are **valid** within the context of the individual's life.

2. Discourage "false starts" with exercise, even consider counseling an individual NOT to begin an exercise program until some of the issues related to their own history and feeling are reviewed. Wait to encourage an individual to begin until they are ready to begin as a lifetime relationship with their bodies versus an activity they "should" do to lose or maintain their weight.

3. Encourage individuals to take 6 months or longer to explore a variety of exercise experiences (consider alternatives such as Yoga, dance, canoeing, bicycling, rollerblading, hiking). During this exploratory period, continue to follow up on how the exercise is experienced. Encourage only situations which are empowering and enjoyable (or potentially enjoyable) to the individual. Discourage dependence on home exercise equipment (boring, novelty wears off), or indoor gym experiences (feelings of futility, inadequacy).

4. Encourage use of exercise trainers ONLY if they are open to learning or understand concepts of exercise for internal reasons NOT to have a more beautiful or even healthy body. Avoid ALL measuring of body fat, anthropometrics, scale weighing, etc.

5. Teach exercise physiology as it relates to aerobic exercise, mitochondria physiology, anaerobic exercise and how both might be experienced by the individual. Avoid encouraging exercising 7 days/ week. Encourage the individual to vary the exercise according to what they discover they enjoy and feel best doing.

Guiding clients toward joyful movement is a gradual process with no formulas. Following are concepts and techniques that can be used with clients. Try these ideas for yourself. Experiment with different strategies. Get the feel of what is suggested. Alter them to better suit your clients' needs. Above all, know that there is not one "right" way to accomplish joyful movement, so enjoy the process!

THE PARADIGM SHIFT

I learned what my body felt like on the inside when it moved and became gradually less concerned with what it looked like on the outside. When I began, sitting on the floor with my legs outstretched, I couldn't even come close to touching my toes. After a month of almost daily practice, I could touch my face to my knees and wrap my hands around my feet. I'd always thought I was inflexible. So much for accurate perceptions about my potential. Anything seemed possible after that.
Tiny seeds of self-acceptance were firmly planted (6).

The chart, Figure 7-C, was adapted from one developed by David Sobel, MD, co-author of *Healthy Pleasures*, highlights a shift from exercise to joyful movement (22).

Figure 7-C   The Shift from Exercise to Joyful Movement

Traditional Exercise	Joyful Movement
* Body Centered Approach	* Mind/Body Approach
* Clinical/Diagnostic Elements	* Clinical/Diagnostic Elements Absent
* Awareness/Fear of Disease Themes	* Experiential/Pleasure Themes
* External Expert/Cue Orientation	* Internal Expert/Cue Orientation
* Competitive Emphasis	* Cooperative Emphasis
* Cultural Conformity Encouraged	* Individual Empowerment Encouraged

---

WORDS OF WISDOM

When helping a client reconnect with joyful movement, always keep in mind:

- Just because a client is large does not mean he or she is exercise resistant. Exercise resistance comes in all shapes, and sizes. These techniques can be used with anyone who has difficulty moving.
- Always work to disconnect activity from "results" such as burning calories, getting rid of fat, body shape, body size, weight, losing weight and/or appearance. Activity may also need to be disconnected from health for some individuals.
- Any exercise with the goal of altering the body, competition or perfection will need to be explored.
- A move must be made to activity with a focus on movement, pleasure, self-fulfillment, social and psychological benefits, energy boosts, and a sense of self-mastery.
- Do not talk about exercise as:

  Cure: "Some extra sit-ups will help get rid of that middle," or "If you exercise, you can have the body you want," or "Two cookies? One mile of walking will take care of that. Don't worry about it."

  Punishment: "Walk an extra mile to help burn off that brownie," or "After what you ate last week, the gym would be a good idea."

- Do not compliment a client based on physical size or shape. When congratulated for weight loss, what does that mean when weight is regained? Most inevitably do regain and feel worse about themselves as a result. When someone says, "I lost weight" a response could be, "How do you feel about that?" Rather than telling someone that they are shaping up, you might say, "You look more content since you have been exercising."
- Joyful movement should be undertaken in a noncompetitive environment with activities that will nurture self-esteem. Do not concentrate on goals or fitness. The biggest mistake is to push too hard too soon, so a slow and gentle start is important. "Encourage your client not to expect improvement overnight. In fact, don't expect anything (24)."

  My goal is to HAVE NO GOALS for exercise. The only prodding to exercise I want to feel is that which comes from my body itself. Even the idea of trying to increase stamina and endurance-- which of course I could do--I don't find those ideas helpful to me at all these days. I am determined to do this right where I am, with no long-range goals at all--however kindly meant, because I know how literally impossible it is for me to separate goals from judgments and feeling fat. I also think I will get to a point when I will naturally start doing some things which are specifically good for my body (such as more exercise to help my knees), but that will have to come later, after I have learned to trust exercise and myself about exercise again and will do such things without the huge meanings attached, etc. (3).

- When your client is ready to choose an activity, encourage her or him to stick with it long enough to find out if they like it. Going to an exercise class or walking once or twice is not enough time to determine if they will enjoy it. It may take 6 weeks for them to begin seeing and feeling the positive effects of movement.

KNOWLEDGE IS POWER

The more your clients understand the positive impact physical activity will have upon their lives, the more likely they will be to try it. However, education focused upon body shaping, calorie burning and weight loss is part of the problem. Refocus education, and do not just teach. Guide a client while providing knowledge. Present facts in a neutral fashion. Take every opportunity to explore and gradually challenge a client's belief systems. Help them shift their motivations for exercise. Bring them to an appreciation of their body. Following are concepts that help challenge the diet mentality view of exercise.

Gradually bring your client to awareness that:
- relatively moderate physical activity enhances health;
- these activities can be part of everyday life;
- it does not have to be a specific exercise regimen, or involve an exercise prescription;
- fitness dramatically decreases when exercise is suddenly curtailed, and there is minimal loss in fitness when exercise is reduced, but not eliminated.

Encourage your clients to read about health and fitness. Suggest some books from the end of this chapter. Remind them, however, of the wisdom not to believe everything they read. "The experts don't agree, and much of what has been written about fat and health, particularly the information found in diet books, is not only untrue but dangerous (6)." Encourage your client to become an expert on their own body, learn what works for them, and temper that with the information from the experts.

HELP CLIENTS INVENTORY THEIR CURRENT SITUATION

Continually explore and challenge cognitive distortions concerning health, fitness and exercise. Inquire about:

Perceived limitations to increasing their activity level:

No time

No money

Fear of harassment

Physical limitations

Past injuries

Failure mind set

Family members who resent time taken time away

Availability of environmental resources, appropriate location and safety issues:

Is it convenient to ride a bike/walk near the house?

Is there a convenient attractive area to ride/walk?

Is it safe to ride/walk there?

Is the traffic conducive to exercise?

Have they checked into exercise classes, fitness centers and trainers for large individuals? Are they size friendly?

Availability of comfortable clothing:

What clothes do they have to wear?

Are they physically comfortable in these clothes?

Are they emotionally comfortable in these clothes?

Do they know where to buy workout clothes, if they want to?

Availability of any workout equipment, pool, track:

Is it in working order?

Is it conveniently located?

Is it comfortable to use?

Is it possible to make it convenient to use?

What is their favorite equipment?

Exercise videos for large persons, i.e. chair exercises, low impact, lead by large persons.

Know where to rent these videos? Keep them in your office to lend out.

Clients' desired goals and expectations:

What, if anything, motivates them to exercise?

What are their short-term goals?

What are their long-term goals?

Are their goals healthy, realistic and safe?

Your clients' past relationships with exercise:

What has motivated them to exercise in the past?

What were the activities they attempted?

How did they feel when they were doing these activities?

Did their bodies change as a result?

If they indicate changes in body shape or weight, inquire about increased mobility, energy, strength, etc.

Was the activity undertaken in conjuction with a diet?

Did they feel they had enough energy to complete the exercise?

What kinds of feedback did they get from others?

What was their reinforcement to continue the activity?

What did they wear?

Why did they quit?

Additional questions:

What music do they like to listen to while exercising?

What time of day is most convenient?

What time of day are they most likely to continue to exercise?

Will they carry/take water with them? In what?

Are showers available?

How will they pull their hair back (if they do)?

Will they need to wash and blow dry their hair after exercise?

Psychological Preparation for Activity

Clients must get ready for activity, psychologically. Activity can be a selfish venture, something they do for themselves. Your clients may spend their day nurturing others, taking little or no time for themselves. They may feel extreme guilt for taking time for themselves. Explore these issues with your clients. They will eventually need to accept that it is okay to do something good for themselves; that they deserve it. Help them understand that physical activity can give them more energy and improve their mood. They may actually end up giving more to others because they have taken time out for themselves.

Trigger for Emotional Pain

Besides the minor aches and pains that arise as a large person's body adjusts to increased movement, emotional pain can also arise. Lyons and Burgard (6) discuss a dance class that was a big hit at a Radiance Retreat, a weekend get-away for large women. A few women left in the middle of the class and later shared how painful it felt to dance. For them it brought up memories of not being asked to dance as teenagers and being told they were too fat. "This long buried pain was triggered along with the desire to be included (6)." Help your client be prepared for this possibility.

FACILITATING MOTIVATION

Help your clients discover their motivations for movement. Goals of weight loss, body shaping, competition and/or perfection will need to be explored. Find out what intrigues them about the idea of movement. What curiosities, concerns, fantasies they have about movement. Identify motives that have nothing to do with weight, or changing the shape of the body. If the goal is overall health and fitness, what does that mean? Do they want to reduce blood pressure or resting heart rate?

Are their goals realistic? When a client is just starting to move, encourage the use of small, attainable behavioral goals, i.e. "I am going to find one friend with whom I can walk at least once a week," or "I am going to try one new activity in the next 3 months" instead of perpetuating the use of far-reaching, often disappointing goals, i.e. "I am going to walk 5 days a week." (Yes, even this relatively small goal may be too much for someone who is exercise resistant.) By making the goals small and attainable, clients have clear evidence of reaching the goal while feeling more self-confident.

For motivation to last, one needs to find that part of themselves that enjoys the sheer exuberance of being active. True motivation for movement comes from a place deep within. Help your client reconnect with that place.   Make sure doubts, fears and hesitancies are discussed and strategies developed to overcome them.

```
┌─────────────────────────────────────────────────────────────────────┐
│  Figure 7-D                                                           │
│                    Possible Motives to Increase Movement              │
│                                                                       │
│  to be full of energy        improved mood       decreased mental and physical tension │
│  improved mental alertness   pleasure            improved sleep quality               │
│  sense of completion         to have fun         raising good/lowering bad cholesterol │
│  increased self-esteem       to play             lowering blood pressure               │
│  self-fulfillment            to move             speed up metabolism                   │
│  sense of self-mastery       to nurture          connection with people                │
│  to feel more alive                              to get rid of stiffness               │
└─────────────────────────────────────────────────────────────────────┘
```

DOING NOTHING IS AN OPTION

Prescribing no activity is also a counseling strategy. Clients who see exercise as a necessary evil, but who start exercising because they are dealing with food-related issues may benefit from committing to do no activity at all. For many, exercise is part of "the wound." Clients may have significant anger about having been required to exercise, but cover this with their eagerness to do the "right" things: lose weight and become more acceptable in the eyes of society. In these cases, the authors suggest:

- exploring their past relationship with exercise and movement,
- exploring their attitudes towards exercise, joyful movement, moving without the goal of weight loss,
- encouraging them to express their feelings,
- reviewing Francie White's suggestions on page 108-109;
- exploring what they enjoyed about activity in the past and what they did not enjoyed. Ask them to complete some of the following Attitude exercises.

Attitudes About Activity

When clients have difficulty finding reasons to move, or can't remember what it feels like to enjoy movement, ask them to find reasons why others move. These exploration assignments are limited only by the imagination. Some suggestions are to ask your client to (18):

- Interview ten people to determine why they like to exercise.
- Interview ten people to find out if their exercise focus is to move the body or to change the body. Which group seem to enjoy exercise more?
- Watch children play for 30 minutes and journal their observations.
- Discuss with a child why they move, what it feels like, why they can't sit still.
- Play with a child where the child has freedom to move around.
- Read books about people enjoying the freedom and accomplishment of movement.

Process these assignments in session. (Processing means discussing an issue thoroughly from a psycho-therapeutic style of counseling, see Chapter 8).

Getting In Touch With Fears

Your clients may have fears about movement. They may not even be aware of them. Have them list their concerns, fears or anxieties about movement and exercise. Through open-ended discussion, explore this list. What can they do to make movement easier or protect themselves from these fears? They will need to suspend judgment especially if some of the worries seem silly. List specific actions they can take to deal with the fears. A very real concern is comments made by rude and callous people, be prepared to discuss this issue.

Moving With Your Client

Exercising during sessions with clients can be a very effective tool in making them feel more comfortable with activity. Take clients through some stretching exercises and discuss sensations and feelings that arise. Ask them to pay attention to their bodies. What muscles want to be stretched? Do they feel tight anywhere? How would they like to move? Make suggestions on which movements will meet their desires. Have a nutrition therapy or stress management session during a walk. Take the opportunity to explore the effects of the activity, how they feel when they move, do their bodies feel warm? Do they have more energy?

Finding The "Hunger For Movement"

I just don't think it's really possible to be all the way accepting and open about food and just part-way about exercise. I have tried that for a long time, and it does not work for me. I think we need to take back our hunger for exercise and desire for movement the way we are reclaiming our hunger for food (3).

Help your client form a vision for their relationship with physical activity. What do they think about when they move? What do they say to themselves? Often individuals in our culture think about how their bodies are changing and how much weight they are losing. They may calculate the exact number of calories they are burning and what dietary transgressions will be undone by activity. They may berate themselves, noticing jiggly thighs, a double chin, or how their clothes do not fit. Or they may compare themselves to other exercisers, real or imaginary. Explore their thoughts and self-talk. Prepare them to alter these if necessary.

I think that the concept of "legalizing" exercise (and "not exercising") can be used the same as it is for eating! Just the same way we allow ourselves to eat whatever, whenever we want - growing more and more in touch with our bodies' needs - we can allow ourselves to play (my word for "exercise"!) however and whenever we want. And if we're not in the mood, it's no big deal. We don't guilt-trip ourselves, just like we don't guilt-trip ourselves over mouth hunger. I think it takes some good self-talk and attention to get to this point, but we did it for the food! So this should translate very well to the exercise issue (3).

RECONNECTING WITH THAT HUNGER TO MOVE

Clients may believe themselves to be couch potatoes and cannot imagine a hunger for movement, much less remember when they last felt it. Ask them to pay attention to times in the day when they are not moving, i.e. waiting in line, watching TV, trying to fall asleep, riding in a car. Do they find themselves tapping their feet, fiddling with their hair or shifting their weight? Ask them to imagine one of these situations in your office and describe how it feels. The antsy feeling they get is their body saying "move." Explore what types of movement they would like to engage in during those antsy times. Help them get in touch with their physical self (6).

What Did I Say?

Ask your clients to take a tape recorder with them when they exercise, saying aloud those things they say to themselves or what they think. Listen to the recording at a session and process what was said. Ask what part of them said (felt) the various comments? Were they talking in 1st or 3rd person, and what was the significance? What feelings drove the comments? Following is a case study illustrating the value of self-talk during exercise:

Janet is a 48 year old paralegal. She has a long history of dieting and is about 100 pounds above her desired weight. As a child and adolescent she was very active in sports and played well, "in spite of my size." She has been in nutrition therapy for six months exploring issues around food, weight and physical activity. She has not participated in any physical activity for the past 20 years, but now feels ready to explore different types of movement. She is starting to walk.

We explored her experience with walking. Did she feel comfortable and safe? Was it how she pictured or was it different? She reported "It was fine." This response always leaves me wanting to know more, and so I inquired about her feelings and thoughts during the activity. She revealed that she yelled at herself. This manifested as loud shouts and words she does not normally use. She was extremely critical and abusive. We explored the issues. Who else has said these things to her? Is this abusive voice in the first person or is it an "outsider's" (intruder's) voice addressing her? She identified that it was primarily an intruder's voice.

I stood up and invited her to come with me. We proceeded out the door and walked for the 30 minutes remaining in the session. For the next four weeks, half of each session was dedicated to the practice of Janet speaking to herself kindly and gently while walking. She had difficulty with this, but she was receptive with guidance. She added compliments and admiration to her self-talk during her walks. Janet finds it difficult to believe the positive comments, but she is beginning to see that it is the negative self-talk that makes exercise so difficult. It is a great improvement over the totally negative talk that used to flood her head. Walking has become somewhat easier for her. Nancy King

Strength And Power
To replace negative self-talk and thoughts, work with your clients to develop visualizations of movement as a way of taking care of themselves such as:
- growing stronger
- arms and legs becoming powerful
- strengthening heart
- strengthening bones
- revving up the engine
- reframing sensations in the body...hot, sweaty, breathless are signals that the body works.

For instance, if walking has been selected:Talk through these visualizations. What would each look like in your clients' minds-eye. Take the opportunity to educate, explain how exercise impacts each of these situations. Be concrete. Discuss how they can use these different visualizations during physical activity.

Conceptualizing Activity in Real Life
Often, clients cannot conceptualize how physical activity will fit in their lives. Talk clients through the specifics of their chosen activity to visualize what they will be doing:

- where will they walk,
- with whom,
- at what time,
- what will they wear,
- how will they make time; who will take care of the kids?
- what will they do when it rains; can they incorporate a walk when they shop at the mall?

If playing ball with a child is the activity planned: when, where, with what ball, what time of day? These in-depth discussions become a type of visualization that helps clients see activity as a part of their week, and eventually, as part of their life.

Exercising To Move The Body Versus To Change The Body
Differentiate between exercise used to "move the body" and that used to "change the body." Exercise resistance and eating disorders are typically fueled when changing the body is the goal. Ask your client to select two physical activities, one with a goal changing the body, the second with a goal of moving the

body. What is their attitude towards these different activities? Ask that they engage in these activities and keep a journal about their experience. Another assignment that works well asks clients to make two lists: one of exercises they believe would change their bodies, and the other, activities that focus on movement. Again, process in session.

Before and After

In our culture, "before" pictures are usually fat and homely and "after" are usually thin and pretty. To help move away from this focus and to help find enjoyment, ask clients to compare, and possibly note in their journal about their mind and body state before and after exercise. Focus on how movement feels before, during and after the activity. Clients record their activity, its duration, and the time of day. Next they can rank the activity on several parameters such as stress level before, during and after the exercise. Often when a person is not looking forward to exercise, he or she feels better once it is accomplished. It is helpful for clients to see this over time. Note how they are feeling during the activity. If a client is not feeling comfortable and positive, make sure to discuss this. Your client may need to pursue another activity. If clients are not exercising for any reason, take the opportunity to check to see how their bodies feel with no exercise.

Rank Impact of Exercise

Ask your clients to record the impact of activity on various physical, emotional and medical parameters for several weeks. Clients should add other information to their journals about the activity's impact on: their stress level, energy level, sense of well-being, sense of empowerment, sense of connection with their body, sense of accomplishment, groundedness and sleep. Use the completed form to explore the impact of movement on your client's life.

Do Not Have Enough Time

If your clients feel they don't have enough free time to be more active, help them reevaluate priorities. If they decide not to pursue activity at this time, work with them to accept the consequences of their choice without judging it. If they intend to play ball or go for a walk but continue to be overwhelmed by life, ask them to schedule two or three 10 minute breaks in their week and commit to them. Have them write these into their appointment book. Process in session.

Positive Comments

Two months ago, I bought a tape, "Yoga for Round Bodies," and experimented. Loved the non competitive atmosphere and the gentle, accepting affirmations the two instructors used: Accepting your present body's limitations and not going further than your body can handle. Emphasized being a C student. After two weeks, on and off, I stopped. Why? Bizarre Behavior Thoughts (BBT) struck. No sweat, no groaning, no pain, no bad body thoughts being pushed by instructors (Remember, "tone that flab," "tighten those buns," "burn that fat"). This wouldn't do. I couldn't be a C student. I wanted that A. [I] wanted to exercise. [I] felt guilty for enjoying myself (3).

Encourage the use of affirmations during exercise such as:
> "I feel my strength when I move."
> "I like myself and feel easy in my body."
> "I am stoking my engine (muscles)."
> "I am a powerful person."
> "I am strong and capable."
> "My body is strong and capable."

Joyful Movement in Private

Locate classes devoted to large women. Check with local large-size clothing stores for men and women, the local YMCA or YWCA, local health clubs, as well as the Yellow Pages under "Health," "Exercise," or "Dance." Look for flyers, ask around. Check with the local NAAFA chapter. Suggest ethnic dance classes, yoga, Tai Chi, and so on. Groups of large individuals could rent exercise space for private exercise classes and avoid rude comments and stares. For instance, a group could share the expense of renting a pool for a couple hours in the morning (a pool with stairs, not just ladders), or they could get together and move to an exercise video.

I got a flier in the mail that announced an introductory class just for "large" women. It said,"Take a walk down the path of self-acceptance while enjoying a lively and fun dance movement class. Experience the camaraderie of being active with other large women." So I went to check it out. ...there's just something wonderful about being surrounded by women my own size. I can feel their support and their acceptance. And I don't fear their disapproval. I can just get into the experience of moving and creating and expressing. Being with other large women in a class like this is so comfortable--it feels like I've come home (25).

Dealing with All or Nothing

Some clients may fear if they quit exercising, they will not go back to it. They are not free to choose whether they want to exercise, they have no choice, they have to exercise. Often these clients follow a daily rigid exercise regimen. They are trapped in an obsession with exercise. They are always focused on the thing (activity) rather than themselves. Work with them to shift the focus to themselves. Explore and discern what are the real reasons clients are afraid they would not go back to exercise. Often they are engaged in a program they do not enjoy, and if they had a choice, they would skip it.

Exercise Abuse...A Cautionary Note

I decided to try to add activity TOTALLY unrelated to what I used to do, which was to go to a health club and do aerobics every lunch hour and swim a mile each evening, until I had chronic pain in my body. I started by walking around my neighborhood, which is safe and has a few gentle hills to challenge myself if I want to. The walking doesn't trigger my exercise fanaticism as much. I can do what feels comfortable, and I don't constantly compare myself now to my old self (3).

Most people think those who abuse exercise are lean individuals that exercise so much they maintain a low percent of body fat. While this is often true, the stereotype overlooks those large individuals who get locked into compulsive exercise. Unfortunately, they are often congratulated on their dedication while the true nature of their unhealthy relationship with exercise is overlooked. Know the signs and symptoms of compulsive exercise, see Figure 7-E, and be prepared to counsel clients through this destructive activity. *Nutrition Therapy* discusses specific techniques to deal with exercise abuse (18).

Figure 7-E   **Symptoms of Exercise Addiction** (26)

- Need to exercise daily to maintain basic level of functioning.
- Express minor withdrawal symptoms (irritability, guilt, anxiety) when unable to exercise for a day or two.
- Experience major withdrawal symptoms (depression, loss of self-esteem, lack of interest in other activities) when unable to exercise for longer periods of time.
- Exercise even against medical advice.
- Risk physical injury.
- Deny pain.
- Organize life around exercise.
- Put exercise above everything else, including job or relationships.
- Strive for greater achievement, no matter how fit or healthy.

SUMMARY

While ideas are endless, the goal is to bring the client to an awareness of joy of movement. Many have never experienced the joyful pleasure and sense of self-mastery as an adult that can come with moving. Reconnecting with this experience is at the core of overcoming exercise resistance.

They're connected. Diet/exercise are like two sides of a coin. How we've learned to value our self-worth. If you change the face value of one side from dieting to feeding, but leave the other intact, still reading exercise as meaning, "bodily or mental exertion, esp. for the sake of training or improvement" (dictionary definition), you have a counterfeit coin, false self-acceptance. Peace comes when your self-worth reflects feeding your hunger and allowing for play "exercise or action by way of amusement or recreation (11)."

Exercise should be done neither as a punishment for looking bad nor as a necessary evil for looking good. It's a gift you give yourself because you need and deserve it. So start playing to play, instead of to win, and you'll find yourself in a no-lose situation. Dinah Shore once said, "I've never thought of participating in sports just for the sake of exercise, or as a means to lose weight, or because it was a social fad. I really enjoy playing. It's a vital part of my life (18)."

RESOURCES: JOYFUL MOVEMENT

Breaking All the Rules. Nancy Roberts. New York: Penguin Books; 1985.

Size acceptance and exercise. Packed with inspiration and information. No specific exercise program.

Compulsive Exercise and the Eating Disorders. A. Yates. New York, NY: Brunner/Mazel, Inc.; 1992.

This book is a thoughtful analysis of the addictions of compulsive athleticism and eating disorders. The author shows that salvation in western culture has been redefined as getting in shape and being aware of calories.

Exercise Physiology: Energy, Nutrition, and Human Performance. McArdle WD, Katch FI, Katch VL. Philadelphia: Lea & Febiger; 1992.

This exercise physiogy text integrates basic concepts and relevant scientific information to provide the foundation for understanding nutrition, energy transfer, and exercise and training. Relevant to the beginner as well as more advanced practitioner. Great color pictures too.

Full Figure Fitness. Bonnie D. Kingsbury. Champaign, Illinois: Life Enhancement Publications; 1988.

Helpful ideas on teaching exercise to large people. Large size models demonstrated exercises. Covers basic concerns for starting a class. Conservative ideas on obesity and health.

Great Shape: The First Fitness Guide for Large Women. Lyons P, Burgard D. Palo Alto, CA: Bull Publishing; 1990.

This excellent book was written directly to large women who may or may not already be involved in physical activity. Both authors, large women themselves, use their personal experience along with professional knowledge to discuss common issues, concerns and anxieties common to want to move their bodies. Practical advise is given in this easy to read book. Professionals would also be well advised to read this book.

Healthy Pleasures: Why Kill Yourself To Save Your Life? Ornstein R, Sobel D. New York, NY: Addison-Wesley Publishing Company; 1989.

Guess what? Exercise is not the only thing that can save your life. Sobel outlines why living a pleasurable life (read: having lots of pleasure in life) can make one healthier...going to a good movie for a laugh, having a glass of wine, petting the dog. He provides research to back up his recommendations.

Hooked on Exercise. Prussin, R. Harvey, P. and DiGeronimo, T. New York: Fireside/Parkside - Simon & Schuster; 1992.

A look at compulsive exercise from a therapists viewpoint. Various functions of compulsive activity are explored and the reader is invited to explore their underlying motivations; i.e. to try to alleviate depression, or to try to improve body image, etc.

Making it Big. Jean du Coffe and Sherry Suib Cohen. New York: Simon and Schuster; 1980.

Discusses large women with exercise and provides a specially designed calisthenics program. Large models are used for demonstrating the exercises, some exercises are hazardous for larger bodies. No aerobics.

The Exercise Fix. Benyo, R. Champaign, IL: Leisure Press; 1990 (139 p).

The story of a runner's compulsive need for the next workout and how it came before family, friends and work. This "reformed runner" takes the reader on a fascinating journey as he describes how a "positive addiction" can turn into a negative addiction, and, with a great deal of work and support, back into a "positive addiction." Helpful for the compulsive exercisers who feel alone in their addiction.

The Gifted Figure: Proportioning Exercises for Large Women. Ann Smith. Santa Barbara: Capra Press; 1984.

Stretches for bigger bodies, large models, emphasis on pleasure and body fitness rather than weight loss. Exercise is inspired by dance and yoga vs cardiovasular fitness. Some stretches are hazardous. Is a good supplement to an exercise program.

The NEW Our Bodies, Ourselves. Boston Women's Health Collective, New York: Simon and Schuster; 1984.

Covers all areas of women's health, including exercise; disabled women, older women, fat women. Gives permission to have fun moving, entitles women the right to be physically active in spite of our culture.

REFERENCES

1. Gavin, J. *The Exercise Habit*. Champaign, IL: Leisure Press; 1992.
2. Author GF. *Radiance: The Magazine For Large Women.* 1993, Winter: 38-42.
3. Overcoming Overeating Internet List-Serve On-going communication between Dec 1995 and Feb 1996.
4. White F, White T. Treating Overweight and Emotional Eating Disorders. Santa Barbara, CA: Handouts From Workshop; September, 1994.
5. Hayes D. Moving Your Body, Feeding Your Body, Loving Your Body. *Hlthy Wt J.* 1995; 9 (2):35-36.
6. Lyons P, Burgard D. *Great Shape: The First Fitness Guide for Large Women.* Palo Alto, CA: Bull Publishing; 1990.
7. Pate RR, Pratt M, Blair SN, Haskell WL, et al. Physical activity and public health: A recommendation fro the Centers for Disease Control and Prevention and the American College of Sports. *JAMA.* 1995; 273: 635-644.
8. Barlow CE, Kohl HW, Gibbons LW, Blair SN. Physical fitness, mortality and obesity *Int J Obes.* 1995; 19: 541-544.
9. Tremblay A, Depres JP, Maheux J, Pouliot MC, Nadeau A, Moorjani S, Lupien PJ, Bouchard C. Normalization of the metabolic profile in obese women by exercise and a low fat diet. *Med and Sci Sports Exerc.* 1991; 23: 1326-1331.
10. Krotkiewski, et al. Effects of long-term physical training on body-fat, metabolism and blood pressure in obesity. *Metabolism.* 1979; 28:650-658.
11. Carrier KM, Steinhardt MA, Bowman M. Rethinking traditional weight management programs: A 3-year follow-up evaluation of a new approach. *J Psych.* 1993; 128(5):517-535.
12. Davis C, Fox J, Cowles M, Hastings P, Schwass K. The functional role of exercise in the development of weight and diet concerns in women. *J Psychosom Res.* 1990;34:563-574.
13. Imm PS, Pruitt J. Body shape satisfaction in female exercisers and non-exercisers. *Women Health.* 1991; 17:53-62.

14. Epling WF, Pierce WD. Activity based anorexia: A bio-behavioral perspective. *Int J of Eating Disord.* 1990; 7:475-485

15. Yates A. *Compulsive Exercise and The Eating Disorders: Toward an Integrated Theory of Activity.* New York: Brunner/Mazel; 1991.

16. American College of Sports Medicine. *Guidelines for Exercise Testing and Prescription.* Philadelphia: Lea & Febiger; 1992.

17. Braith RW, Graves JE, Pollock ML, Lggett SL, Carpenter DM, Colvin AB. Comparison of two versus three days per week of variable resistance training during 10 and 18 week programs. *Int J of Sports Med.* 1989; 10:450-454.

18. Kratina KM. "Exercise Resistance, Compulsion and Recommendations." In: Helm K, Klawitter B, Eds. *Nutrition Therapy: Advanced Counseling Skills.* Lake Dallas, TX: Helm Seminars; 1995.

19. Ernsberger P. Heavy breathing for health. *Radiance: The Magazine For Large Women.* 1988; 80:37-39.

20. Ornstein R, Sobel D. *Healthy Pleasures.* New York, NY: Addison-Wesley Publishing Company;1989.

21. White F, White T. Treating Overweight and Emotional Eating Disorders. Santa Barbara, CA: Handouts From Workshop; September, 1994.

22. Sobel, D. Healthy Pleasures: Why Kill Yourself to Save Your Life. Las Vegas, NV: Handouts from presentation: New World Fitness IDEA 1994 Convention, Las Vegas;1994.

23. Freedman, R. *BodyLove: Learning to Like Our Looks and Ourselves.* New York: Harper & Row; 1989.

24. Rich SL. Hey Sis - an exercise class just for us! *Radiance: The Magazine For Large Women.* 1993; Fall: 14-15, 40.

25. Omichinski L, Harrison KR. *Nondiet Weight Management: A Lifestyle Approach to Health & Fitness.* San Marcos, CA: Nutrition Dimension; 1995.

8

Communicating the Concepts

> *Attentive care fosters self-regard, self-protection, and self-control. Having one's needs met fosters a view of the world as responsive and caring, which in turn leads to self-regulation and a sense of equilibrium and well-being* (1).

ADVISING OR GUIDING?

Counseling is defined by Webster's Dictionary as "to give advice or guidance (2)." Most health care professionals are trained in college to give advice. In fact, that is the traditional medical model. Originally, dietitians were taught to fill out a meal plan and provide a 20 to 30-minute diet consultation based on diagnosis prior to a patient's discharge from a hospital. Fitness professionals use this approach when they design an exercise prescription based on the results of an objective fitness test. Physicians make a diagnosis, prescribe a treatment and give advice. Giving advice is much more specific and time-efficient than providing a client with guidance. However, research suggests that guidance, *rather than advising*, is actually more effective in helping people change lifestyle habits.

This author recalls her first job as a clinical dietitian. I was asked to provide a diet instruction to a 43 year old female with insulin dependent diabetes who was 100 pounds over her ideal body weight. We spent an hour reviewing her 1,200 calorie diabetic exchange list diet. Most of my clients met me with a big smile, asked several questions, and basically affirmed that they would live their new lifestyle; I always had my doubts. My doubts came to life in this woman's despair and anguish as she recounted never being able to accurately follow a diet, and not sure she could do it at this time either. I cried when I left that session, knowing my efforts had been ineffective, but worse, not knowing what else I could do to help this woman.

Finding and developing a new style of counseling took many years. During the transition, I counseled a 45 year old male who had made some basic changes in his eating and exercise styles, but he continued to drink 4 to 12 beers every night. Since he did not see this as a problem, I didn't think it would work to tell him to quit drinking or to cut back. I did realize, however, that somehow it had to be his idea. I asked open-ended questions, explored his relationship with alcohol and challenged the assumptions he had about his relationship with alcohol. I knew what I wanted him to do, but he seemed to be unaware of my agenda. As we continued to explore the options, he suddenly looked at me in surprise and said, "You know, this beer drinking is really getting in my way." I affirmed that I thought that he probably was right. He suggested maybe he would cut down his intake of beer.

Over the years I found eliciting information from clients was much more effective than providing advice on the proper diet. My experiences taught me that using the medical model of therapy for nutrition or lifestyle counseling fosters minimal success rates with clients compared to a more interactive style where clients help explore the problems and develop their own solutions. Karin Kratina

DEVELOPING A PSYCHOTHERAPEUTIC STYLE OF COUNSELING

In order to move into a psychotherapeutic style of counseling, most traditionally trained health care professionals need additional skills. In guidance-oriented counseling, health care providers meet with clients over a longer period of time, encountering the more complicated dynamics of extended therapeutic relationships. Unfortunately, many are not prepared to deal effectively with this type of counseling (3). Instead, they use a medical model which involves:

- short-term intervention primarily of an educational nature,
- a minimal relationship,
- a quickly determined, often standardized plan of action.

This approach works when education of the person is the primary objective (3). By contrast, a psychotherapeutic model involves:

- long term care,
- a significant relationship that in and of itself is a key part of the therapeutic process,
- a treatment plan that is highly individualized and evolves over time.

Some experts believe that for health care providers to become proficient in working with eating problems as well as self-acceptance and exercise resistance, they must develop psychotherapeutic skills (3).

Professional Supervision

Typically, it is psychotherapists and mental health counselors who are trained in the psychotherapeutic model. They are required to be involved in at least a year of professional supervision of skills and receive ongoing feedback to improve therapeutic strategies and techniques. Additionally, supervision helps them identify personal issues which, untouched, can interfere with the therapeutic process.

Health care providers involved in counseling can also benefit from professional supervision. Supervision from a therapist, dietitian, or other professional skilled in the psychotherapeutic model can be extremely helpful while developing this style of counseling. Supervision, which involves discussion and review of case studies, helps you understand and deal with issues such as denial, manipulative behavior, power struggles, and counter transference that may arise in long-term work with clients.

Professional supervision can be accomplished 1:1 or in group settings. One-on-one supervision allows more time to explore individual cases and more opportunity to explore personal issues. Group supervision allows the opportunity for several professionals to meet, discuss cases, and share experiences. The group may share the expense and have a skilled therapist facilitate the group occasionally or on an ongoing basis (4). The fee charged for supervision is usually similar to what therapists charge clients.

Learn About Counseling From The Client's Perspective

Many health care providers have found it invaluable to experience the counselor/client relationship first hand as a client. To do this, locate a therapist whose work you respect and commit to a specific time period of therapy. Assess your own relationship with food, weight, exercise, body image, and size acceptance. Discover what techniques, approaches, and counseling styles you prefer. Keep a personal journal. Learn to be able to identify, talk about, write about and express your feelings (5).

Referring Clients to Other Professionals

Large individuals will often need to be referred for medical care if they have a medical condition or they plan to significantly increase their activity level. Be careful when referring out. Make sure the physician, dietitian, exercise counselor, psychotherapist, physical therapist, and other professionals are size friendly. It is the referring clinicians' responsibility to send large clients to other practitioners who do not shame them, blame their condition on weight, or admonish them to lose weight. See Chapter 2 for questions a clinician or client may ask to find size friendly health providers. Following is an example of a psychotherapist who treats eating problems, but "doesn't get it," and should be avoided.

Robbie is a professional woman and mother who, at 5'6", weighs 235#. She and her husband recently met with a psychotherapist for brief marital counseling. The therapist is a well-known specialist in the field of eating disorders. At the end of the first session (a session in which Robbie nor her husband brought up her weight), the therapist said as they were walking out the door, "Have you ever thought about dropping some weight." An embarrassed Robbie explained she has tried over and over and of course she would like to lose weight. The therapist then recommended she try one of the new anti-obesity drugs. When Robbie said she did not want to resort to drugs, the therapist suggested she eat salad before each meal to dull her appetite. The therapist went so far as to suggest that Robbie take the salad to work and have it about 1 hour before lunch. What is wrong with this picture?

Working With a Therapist or a Treatment Team

Sometimes those with eating problems and exercise resistance work with several different professionals at the same time. More often, the client's health care providers will find themselves inadequately prepared to deal with all of the medical and psychological issues that arise and will need to refer their client to other professionals. For instance, a psychotherapist may refer to an exercise physiologist to help reframe cognitive distortions regarding exercise. A dietitian may refer a client with bulimia to a dentist to deal with enamel erosion.

Continuing collaboration with all members of the treatment team will increase effectiveness with clients. Establish boundaries with other team members. Determine mutual responsibilities of treatment. What happens when the client asks the therapist a nutrition-related question? When working with a treatment team there is potential for "splitting," a situation in which the client pits one member of the team against another. Effective communication helps avert this (6). Maintain contact with other team members, either by making an appointment to talk in person or by phone, with brief progress notes, or by leaving a message on the therapists voice mail (make sure it is a confidential line). You may want to set up a standard meeting time, possibly at lunch. This is ideal if you have several clients in common (6).

New Resources

To further improve counseling style, read books that discuss assertiveness, getting in touch with feelings, and so on. Take an advanced psychology class to learn about different counseling styles, nutrition, exercise, esteem issues and other psychological concerns (i.e. personality disorders, specific treatment intervention, and so on). Attend conferences that can expand your skills. Find out from local psychologists, social workers, mental health counselors, dietitians, exercise physiologists or other appropriate professionals what resources and workshops are available. Conferences on eating disorders frequently explore counseling, nutrition, exercise, and psychological issues that are useful to health care professionals in everyday practice (6).

The need for increased skills is becoming more widely recognized. For instance, two different groups have formed within The American Dietetic Association to promote this form of counseling: the Disordered Eating Networking Group within the Sports and Cardiovascular Nutritionists (SCAN) Practice Group; and the Nutrition Therapists within the Nutrition Entrepreneurs (NE) Practice Group. Contact your professional organization for further information. The Association for the Health Enhancement of Large Persons, the National Eating Disorders Organization, the International Association of Eating Disorder Professionals, and The Renfrew Foundation Conference have yearly conferences where professionals of all backgrounds are welcome. They have presentations that help improve the skill level of the neophyte as well as the more seasoned professional. (See resources on page 149 for more information on these organizations.)

An in-depth discussion of psychotherapeutic counseling skills is beyond the scope of this manual. Reading available literature is highly recommended. An excellent compilation of psychotherapeutic nutrition counseling strategies and techniques is available in *Nutrition Therapy* (7). The reference list has other resources.

ENHANCING THE COUNSELING PROCESS
Connecting with others not only enhances one's mental health,
but physical health and recovery as well (8).

At the heart of guiding your client to a healthier lifestyle is connecting or establishing a relationship with them. Study after study shows that those who have a sense of belonging or closeness to a person or group have a greater sense of well-being, recover from physical trauma faster and live longer after life-threatening illnesses (8). It can be assumed that health professionals who foster a sense of connection with their clients, especially when discussing emotionally-charged issues such as food and weight, will have a greater positive impact on their clients (8). Dean Ornish, in *Reversing Heart Disease* (9) sums it up with, "In short, anything that promotes a sense of isolation leads to chronic stress and often to illnesses like heart disease. Conversely, anything that leads to real intimacy and feelings of connection can be healing."

To make use of the healing power of connection, you must be able to bond with the client, but the client must also feel connected to you. Following are some basics of connection. As you read over them, assess your own ability to provide an environment where you can connect with your client.

- Provide support in the form of undivided, unbiased attention. Not only must you be supportive, you must look supportive. This support will enhance rapport and help build clients' self-esteem. Clients who believe in themselves are better able to make necessary lifestyle changes. This kind of support also helps clients deal more honestly with themselves, rather than feel a need to hide in fear, shame or anger. Basically, the more you accept them, the more they can accept themselves.

- Be fully receptive. Do you know, almost intuitively, when a person is only half-listening to you? What does that feel like? How distracting is it for you when you are trying to discuss an important issue with someone, and they are playing with a pencil, shaking a leg, playing with their hair or zoning out? Fully commit to interactions with your clients, and be receptive with emotions, words, and body signals. Have you ever talked to somebody and know instantly that they do not believe you? How do you know that they don't believe you? Do you do this with your clients?

MOVING BEYOND THE SYMPTOMS
A woman who starts treatment talking about her food obsession may be revealing her
deepest intimate needs and her psychic organization (10).

For most individuals, food and body image issues have deeply personal meanings. These meanings differ from person to person, and significantly influence eating and exercise patterns. Clients can be assisted in changing their eating and exercise patterns through the exploration of their relationship with food and with their bodies. Through this exploration, the health care provider can begin to decode the clients' eating, exercise and weight-related experiences. Psychotherapeutic counseling skills are needed to move through this process; however, always be aware of and work within the scope of your practice.

Body focus, weight obsession, dieting, and dysfunctional exercise *(these are all examples of symptoms of eating problems)* can all function to keep clients from experiencing and examining certain feelings, thoughts, conflicts, identifications, needs, and fantasies. At the same time, the symptom expresses these same feelings, identifications, and so forth (10). These symptoms can be used as a defense to thoughts and feelings the client finds uncomfortable or troublesome and wants to avoid. These symptoms can actually function in such a way as to block awareness of anything except the symptom (weight, food, etc.). These symptoms can defend against certain feelings (e.g. anger) or push away particular experiences.

Severity of Symptoms

...the addictive power of the diet does not lie only in its value as a relief fantasy. The actual experience of dieting creates addicts. As one engages in the diet, the need to diet is re-created and enforced (10).

The range in severity of symptoms associated with the dieting mentality is significant. The majority of individuals who diet are not totally "taken over" by their symptoms and obsessions, yet. There is a preoccupation that changes in intensity, depending on what is going on in their lives. For these individuals, it serves to modulate anxiety, need states and esteem (10).

There are others for whom the symptom substitutes for life itself. The focus of every single day is activity (mental and physical) in the service of eating or not eating, running, sneaking, bingeing. For these individuals, the defenses and symptoms act as a safeguard against greater anxiety, disintegration, and fear of exposing their neediness to themselves and to others, thereby leaving them less open to rejection and abandonment (10).

Exploring Adaptive Functions of the Symptom

You can learn a great deal from the client through the process of detailed questioning about food and weight related behaviors. Carefully chosen questions can help the client begin to see that another way of thinking exists. Open-ended questions allow the opportunity for the client to experience feelings and reflect upon them. As the clients see the problem is not weight or their bodies, they often experience a sense of relief from feelings of inadequacy and failure.

For example, one client, Brenda, reported she was extremely bored with food. Exploration revealed that this boredom was actually displaced anger, but not at the food, she was angry with the treatment team. She defended herself from feelings by shifting those feelings to food. Once this was identified, she was better able to explore and make changes in her eating patterns. Brenda was referred to her psychotherapist to discuss these feelings in more depth.

The clinician must realize clients' relationship with food and weight is highly symbolic. You may find when talking about food, eating, weight, and exercise with clients, they are quickly taken to the essence of their emotional experience. Even their difficulties talking about it tell a story (10). These discussions may help to reveal what might have remained unavailable.

The Client's Story

To understand a symptom or an aspect of it, the health care provider must first slow down the client's rapid presentation by asking for a more detailed account of the eating, exercise, or negative body thought experience. This detailed accounting is absolutely essential. Clients usually tell the story quickly with full focus on the final destination: self-blame and self-recrimination. Self-blame often masks or hides major psychological issues that cannot be dealt with and integrated if continually bypassed by focusing only on the blame (10). It is therefore important for the health care provider to slow down the story telling in order to explore each aspect of it. It is in this slowing down that the psychological purpose of the thought or action can be revealed. This is essential if the goal is more than symptom removal.

DECODING THE SYMPTOM

All the following are prominent metaphors in the symbolic language of women with eating problems. They must be treated as metaphors for a persistent, gnawing, emotional hunger that will not subside no matter what food or exercise strategy is employed. The seemingly garbled code of their images, action, and thoughts must be deciphered (10). Decoding means (2) to convert the code into intelligible language.

- heading straight for the diet/health section of the bookstore;
- thinking of food before anything else each morning;
- covering leftovers with salt;
- attacking one's body curves by exercising for 6 hours (10);
- obsessive thinking and over involvement with the body (10);

- repeatedly eating with no regard for the body's signals of hunger and satiety;
- conversations that center around the latest diet and pounds lost.

Approach each discussion of food, exercise, and weight-related behavior with a stance of compassion, curiosity, empathy and attention. It is essential to avoid judging the client while you maintain an open, questioning attitude. In the face of the patient's great shame or trivialization of the problem, the therapist must create a safe place in which the problem can be articulated, dignified, and eventually worked through. The very process of detailed inquiry into eating behavior and the feelings that trigger and accompany it dignifies the symptom by making it worthy of serious psychological investigation. Therapists need to communicate tolerance for the symptom itself, for the intensity of feelings, as well as for the symbolic content of the symptom (10). This can be done by bringing the symptom into the therapeutic dialogue with empathy and curiosity.

Josie was a 19 year old woman who began her first diet at age 12 and came to believe that 1,200 calories was more than adequate. She joined several commercial weight loss programs where she lost the same 10 pounds but always dropped out. By 16, she regularly engaged in deprivation-driven binge eating while trying to maintain a 1,200 calorie diet. Within a year she was purging by vomiting and with laxatives. At age 18 she began to see a therapist. She discussed her behavior on a superficial level quite easily and did so repeatedly. As the therapist began to delve further into the behavior, she no longer discussed it easily. It was clear that she felt much guilt and shame about the purging behavior. She also felt out of control during these episodes and was terrified of revisiting these feelings. She became less communicative and avoided the issues. The therapist pursued the topic in a manner that would normalize the behavior to help reduce shame, explaining the use of the symptom helped Josie survive when she had few other coping skills. To help normalize the behavior, she asked detailed questions about the purging episodes, "Josie, I'm wondering if you could tell me a little about your purging so I might understand it better. For instance, I once had a client who always used a specific hair ribbon to pull her hair out of her face and another who would always start a binge with tomato juice. It was a kind of marker so that she would know when she had brought up all the food in the binge. I'm wondering if you have any specific rituals, do you put on music, leave the water running. All these parts of the purge are messages we can decode. Do you think we can talk about a few of these?"

The often repetitive manner in which the eating and exercise incidents and negative body thoughts are presented can belie the profound and varied meanings contained therein. It may seem as though there is no need to pursue the details of the incidents further, believing you have heard one, you have heard them all. However, in an effort to decode and move beyond the symptom, the clinician must listen carefully to the content with an attitude of fresh curiosity.

The goal of decoding a symptom is not necessarily to avoid the symptom. Rather the process is intended to heighten the client's awareness of a compulsion to engage in the specific behavior. Awareness provides a basis for choice:

1) notice the symptom and use it to get in touch with feeling or needs;
2) choose to continue to use the symptom in an attempt to address the feeling or meet the need, albeit ineffectively.

Decoding a food or weight related thought or behavior is part of empowering a client to move beyond the thought or behavior, and eventually beyond the symptom.

THE IMPORTANCE OF FEELINGS

Not to be aware of one's feelings, not to understand them or know how to use or express them is worse than being blind, deaf or paralyzed. Not to feel is not to be alive (11).

In order to successfully decode eating and exercise problems, it is imperative that you are able to identify, tolerate and discuss feelings, both your own and your client's. Many individuals find it uncomfortable to deal with feelings, which is why we so often see the use of food (alcohol, drugs, work, smoking, etc.) to avoid them. Those with eating and exercise problems specifically use food or exercise to defend against feelings. When feelings are avoided this way, there is continued need to use the substance. It is only when the feelings are addressed and your client can deal with them appropriately that they can make the changes they desire.

Know Your Own Feelings

To help clients move beyond diets successfully, you must be able to deal with your own feelings. This can be a very uncomfortable process. You may not even know whether you are in touch with your feelings.

Early in my counseling career, I attended a communications-building workshop and filled out a Myers-Briggs Personality Type Indicator Test. As I took the test, it was very obvious to me that answers on one end of the scale sounded intelligent and only a fool would pick those on the other end. To my surprise, I scored 20 points as a Thinker and 0 points in Feeling style of personality. As I reviewed the questions, those "foolish" answers that I had so little regard for were ones that showed more feeling. I learned a great deal at that workshop. I realized I needed to get in touch with my feelings, but it took years before I could talk about them.

Since identifying, tolerating, and appropriately discussing feelings is such a critical part of this process, some time will be spent exploring these issues. Get involved with and practice the concepts outlined below in order to enhance your skill as a guiding counselor.

In the space below, write a statement about a feeling you experienced within the last 24 hours. Now draw a face that shows that feeling on a blank sheet of paper or use the form provided in the handout packet. We will come back to this in a moment. Figure 8-A on page 128 shows a variety of emotions as interpreted from facial expressions. Use this form to help clients identify their feelings.

Describe a Feeling: _____

_____

_____

Dealing With Feelings

Our feelings summarize what we have experienced and tells us if it is pleasurable or painful (11).

Dealing with your own feelings will help clarify personal issues as well as counter transference issues* that may arise in counseling situations with clients. Helping a client to identify his or her feelings helps to open up communication and enhance trust. Healing eating problems involves identifying and exploring the feelings hidden by the behavior (decoding the symptom) and helping the client find healthier coping strategies. This does not mean that a psychotherapist will be engaging in nutrition therapy or a medical doctor will be engaging in psychotherapy. Health care providers must stay within the scope of their practice. Most can "help the client define problems, accept the client's feelings, [give] permission for normal responses, [expect] the client to handle the problems, and [suggest] specific follow-up assignments and tasks (12).

* Counter transference is when a feeling is invoked in the health care provider as a result of identification with a feeling or experience that the patient may be having. For example, a patient talking about how nobody understands her may evoke feelings of incompetence in the health care provider (13).

Figure 8-A

Feeling Faces

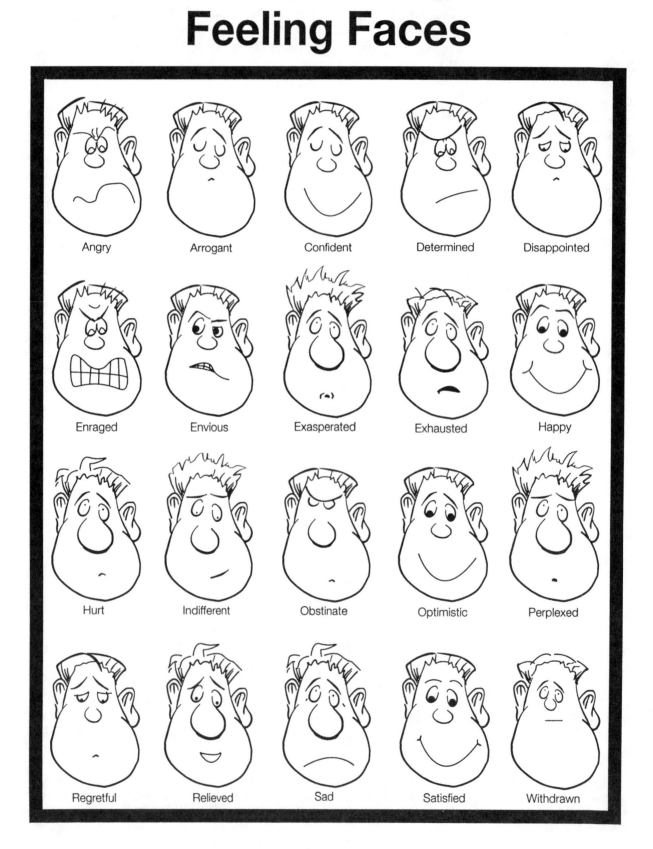

Lifeskills such as identifying and discussing feelings, assertiveness, stress management, maintaining appropriate boundaries and other coping skills can be explored. It is the psychotherapists who delve into such issues as "suicidal tendencies, physical abuse, severe marital difficulties, feelings of depression, past unresolved sexual abuse, recurring self-destructive behaviors (7)," and so on.

No two people perceive an experience the same way, but there are common ways in which we deal with reactions to the experience--feelings. While we each differ in what we think is important, we are very much alike in the way we react to an important event such as loss. Since feeling responses are so universal, we can understand others feelings and have compassion for them. Feelings are the reaction to what we perceive. "When we use words alone to describe what we perceive we are really attempting to manage feelings rather than experience them. Thinking is a much more indirect way of handling reality than feeling. Feelings tell us when something is painful and hurts, because feelings are the hurt. Thought explains the hurt, justifying, rationalizing, putting it into perspective (11)."

If you do not recognize your feelings, you cannot be in touch with what is really going on in your life. Feelings are truth. Using defenses to try to manage feelings may distort your perception of the truth, but it does not alter that truth. Explaining feelings away does not resolve them or exorcise them. They have to be dealt with. Putting the blame on others does not take away feelings, or reduce their intensity. Feelings may be disguised, denied, rationalized, but a painful feeling will not go away until it has run its natural course. In fact when a feeling is avoided, its painful effects are often prolonged and it becomes increasingly difficult to deal with it (11).

Just as physical pain causes us to move away from some danger, when an emotional injury threatens, our natural reaction is to avoid it. If injury is not avoidable, it should be seen as a very real threat, and preparations made to reduce the extent of the threat so a resolution can be found. Sometimes, though, we overreact to painful feelings and set up impenetrable defenses. When our feelings are altered by such defenses, separating us from pain, managing feelings can become difficult because we simply lose sight of the problem (11). The defenses will serve to protect us from further injury; however, when used to shield from all pain, defenses can use so much energy that they have almost the same depleting effect as the injury itself. The energy used for defenses is used to put up and maintain a barrier to reality. Each of us needs to find a balance between pain and defense and rely on his own experience as a guide. While we frequently have little choice whether to use a defense or not, we can lower our defenses by enduring as much pain as we can tolerate until most of the pain is gone. It's not easy, it takes courage, but it works (11).

Learning the Language of Feelings
The language of feelings is the means by which we relate to ourselves, and if we cannot communicate with ourselves we simply cannot communicate with others (11).

Many people use the word "feel" in conversation without ever expressing a feeling. For instance, "I feel like going to the mall," is not a feeling statement; neither is "I feel like you are angry at me." The following discussion should help you to clarify feelings with your clients.
- Using the word "feel" in a sentence, as in "I feel _____," does not necessarily make the sentence an expression of a feeling. For example, "I feel like you don't like me" is not a feeling; it is a thought. "I feel rejected" is a feeling.
- In fact, almost without exception, if a sentence starts with "I feel <u>like</u>...," a *thought* is about to be expressed, *not* a feeling.
- Feelings can always be expressed as one word.
- Likewise, if a group of words is used to express a feeling, it is most likely not a feeling.

The difference between thoughts and feelings is important.
- *When we think about feelings, we attempt to manage them rather than experience them.* Thinking is a much more indirect way of handling reality than feeling. Thoughts explain the hurt, justifying, rationalizing, putting it into perspective Webster's (2) defines thought as "an opinion, viewpoint or belief; a product of thinking: idea."

- Feelings tell us when something is painful and hurts, because feelings are the hurt. We need to fully experience feelings in order to be able to move through them. On the other hand, a feeling is defined as "emotion; a distinct mood or impression; intuitive cognition, hunch (2)."

Another way to clarify feelings is to use the following two rules:
- If "think" can be substituted for "feel" in a sentence, it is *not* a feeling. For instance, consider the comment: "I feel you are overly concerned about the food I am choosing." Substitute the word "think" for the word "feel." "I think you are being overly concerned about the food I am choosing." Since using "think" results in a coherent sentence, this sentence is expressing a thought, not a feeling.
- If "am" can be substituted for "feel," it's a feeling. Consider the following sentence: "I feel angry that you are making comments about the food I am choosing." Substitute "am" for "feel." "I am angry that you are making comments about the food I am choosing." Since "am" can be used, this sentence does express a feeling.

Just to double check, take the last sentence and substitute "think" for "am." "I think angry that you are making comments about the food I am choosing." It doesn't work; the sentence is not a thought, it is a feeling.

There are several words that fit into the above examples, but still do not express feelings. For example, *good* and *bad* are not feelings. "I feel good" does not express a feeling. Webster's Dictionary (2) defines *good* as "having desirable or favorable qualities, appropriate, convenient, beneficial, competent, genuine, pleasant, virtuous, benevolent and loyal." When someone says to you, "I feel good," what is it exactly that they are expressing? We do not get a lot of information from a statement like that. Were they to say, "I feel happy," or "I feel content," or "I feel smug," one would have much more information than from the statement, "I feel good." *Bad* is defined as "poor, inferior, evil, disobedient, unfavorable, decayed (2)." "I feel bad," does not express a feeling. "I feel uncomfortable," or "I feel angry," or "I feel sad," expresses a feeling, and is more telling than the phrase, "I feel bad."

We have all heard the phrase, "I feel fat." Interestingly, fat is also not a feeling. This concept is discussed further on pages 136-139.

Another way to differentiate between thoughts and feelings is to remember that feelings usually, with the above exceptions, can be expressed as one word. If an expression of feelings turns into a string of words, it is probably not a feeling. For instance, "I feel like you don't like me." This is not a feeling. However, if one were to say, "I feel unloved." This is one word and it is a feeling. Checking it with the previous test, "I am unloved," does work, so this is a feeling being expressed.

Review the feeling statement you made on the earlier page. Make sure it is a feeling and not a thought. If a thought is expressed, rework it so that it expresses a feeling. Next, show the drawing to a partner or friend and have him or her guess what feeling is represented. Describe the feeling, using only feeling terms.

The Feeling List, Figure 8-B, can be used to become familiar with naming different feelings. This list can also be used help understand feelings. For instance, your clients may state they feel anxiety when faced with eating at a party. Anxiety is a difficult feeling to comprehend. Why do they feel anxious? For simple clarification purposes, feelings can be loosely divided into 4 groups: afraid, glad, mad and sad. Provide your clients with the Feelings List and ask them to identify under which main feeling anxiety falls. They will find anxiety under "afraid." Anxiety is a type of free-floating fear. You can then explore what fears the client may have about eating at the party. Of course, this may be oversimplifying the feeling or the situation, so make sure you do not negate the intensity or meaning of the originally stated feeling.

Figure 8-B

FEELINGS LIST

AFRAID	GLAD	MAD	SAD
Ambivalent	Amazed	Abused	Abandoned
Anxious	Amused	Aggressive	Agonized
Apprehensive	Calm	Alienated	Apologetic
Bewildered	Cherished	Angry	Burdened
Cautious	Comfortable	Apathetic	Desperate
Confused	Confident	Appalled	Disappointed
Cowardly	Content	Blamed	Discouraged
Disoriented	Determined	Bitter	Disregarded
Fearful	Delighted	Bored	Distant
Frantic	Eager	Controlled	Embarrassed
Frightened	Ecstatic	Disapproving	Empty
Hesitant	Exhilarated	Disgusted	Foolish
Insecure	Free	Enraged	Forgotten
Panicked	Fulfilled	Envious	Grief
Paranoid	Happy	Exasperated	Hopeless
Perplexed	Hopeful	Frustrated	Humiliated
Puzzled	Important	Furious	Hurt
Restless	Joyous	Guilty	Hysterical
Scared	Loving	Hostile	Impotent
Suspicious	Loose	Horrified	Isolated
Threatened	Mellow	Impatient	Jinxed
Timid	Mischievous	Indifferent	Lonely
Torn	Nurturing	Irritated	Lost
Uncertain	Optimistic	Lethargic	Miserable
	Peaceful	Manipulated	Neglected
	Playful	Negative	Overlooked
	Protective	Ornery	Regretful
	Proud	Resentful	Rejected
	Relieved	Shocked	Upset
	Respected	Smothered	Withdrawn
	Satisfied	Stubborn	Worthless
	Sympathetic	Victimized	Vulnerable

Moving Away From Diets
Helm Seminars, Publishing (817) 497-3558

The Appropriate/Inappropriate Expression of an Emotion form, Figure 8-C, developed by Francie White, MS, RD, may also be useful with clients (14). Use these forms to explore your own feelings before using them with clients. Discuss your feelings with someone who is skilled at doing this. Supervision is an excellent place to process this work. The books on the reference list are also helpful.

Using Feelings In The Counseling Process

Health care providers who become skilled at expressing and discussing feelings will progress more quickly with their clients. Without this skill you will not be effective in helping clients decode the symptoms of their eating problems or exercise resistance. Ask clients to practice making feeling statements. When they say, "I feel like….," remind them they have just expressed a thought and ask for clarification of the feelings   Clients need to be reminded:

- all feelings are normal,
- there is no such thing as right or wrong feelings, feelings just are,
- it is understandable to be upset with uncomfortable feelings, and
- talk with your counselor about feelings that arise.

As people become more open with their feelings there's less need to guard against things in the world that are threatening; for instead of hiding from feelings, the open person uses them as a guide that interprets the world he is experiencing (11).

Uncomfortable Feelings

In long-term, close relationships with clients, health care professionals are more likely to come across negative emotions, such as anger, hostility and reluctance. Dealing with these emotions effectively seldom is a part of health providers' training. Too often clients are placated, made to feel good, or manipulated into an unthreatening place of neutrality. In other words, rather than dealing with the clients' feelings, health providers' often try to change them, avoid them, or redirect them. While this makes the health care providers more comfortable, it does little for the client except provide some passing relief.

We need to be skilled at dealing with uncomfortable feelings. Since resistant clients usually bring up significant uncomfortable feelings to the health care provider, and often clients are uncomfortable and not in touch with their own feelings, we will explore the feelings issue more closely.

MOVING THROUGH RESISTANCE

When working with a resistant client, it is often helpful to reframe the resistance as reluctance. Resistance implies barriers. Reluctance becomes easier to deal with because it connotes hesitance. Ways in which clients express reluctance will be examined below. We suggest techniques to deal with the reluctance, as well as other feelings.

Reluctance Takes Many Forms

It is helpful to identify reluctance in order to move through it. Following are common ways clients express reluctance:

- silliness, laughing;
- minimal communication: nodding, shrugging, or silence;
- revealing only low-priority items;
- refusal to accept the notion that help is needed;
- over-compliance; eager advice-seeking;
- revealing only what is expected, therapy-wise;
- defensiveness;
- diversionary excursions, e.g. repeatedly telling you the life history of a daughter.

Figure 8-C APPROPRIATE/ INAPPROPRIATE EXPRESSION OF AN EMOTION
by Francie White, MS, RD.   Used with permission.

EMOTION	APPROPRIATE EXPRESSION	INAPPROPRIATE EXPRESSION
Sad	Crying, sobbing, talking & crying = blubbering, rocking, sweating, writing, art, holding still & feeling, telling story (with tears) . . . , spending time on it.	"Being strong", holding in, sulking, manipulating, blaming behavior, avoiding i.e., using addictions instead of feeling, getting mad at everyone else, guilt.
Mad	Concentrating on the feeling, pinpointing its source, confronting, risking losing approval, setting firm boundaries, letting go of being nice, beating on pillows, in-session screaming, yelling, sweating, being loud, writing, setting limits, bottom lines, raging in session, laughing, crying.	Raging (anger with intent to hurt, tear down, destruct another), stuffing, suppressing, chickening out, getting depressed, using addiction, rationalizing, projecting fault & blame in generalized way, moodiness, avoidance.
Fear	Shaking, rocking, fetal position, crying, beating on pillow, talking-telling story. Saying "I'm afraid" over & over. Risking, confronting what needs confronting, sweating. <u>Being held.</u> Laughing.	Avoidance via substance, stuffing, minimizing, being strong, rationalizing. "It's not so bad". Projecting blame to others.
Glad	Stopping and feeling, reveling in feeling, sharing via talking, art, journaling. Pursuing it, more toward, laugh, cry, scream.	Feeling guilt, minimize it, suppress, use substance, not share it, feel unentitled, shame, withdraw, quiet.

Panic is a normal counselor's reaction when you are confronted with these behaviors by a client. ("I feel panicked right now." Look up panicked in the Feelings List. What is the underlying feeling?) The most automatic response is, "What am I doing wrong?," or you may think, "He is really being a pain." If you become impatient, judgmental, angry, or unwilling to accept the clients as they are, as they present themselves, you will not be able to see what's going on in the therapeutic relationship. Clients need to be accepted as they present themselves in order to move through reluctance. In other words, it's okay for the client to be reluctant. But then how do you deal with these feelings?

Pay Attention to The Reluctance
Check your own reaction.
Do not take reluctance personally. Note your own reaction and feelings. Note whether you take it personally, or if it creates uncomfortable feelings. Reframe what is happening so it is not about you, but about the client. One way to do this is to say to yourself. "Isn't this fascinating? Mary Jane is sneering at me; I wonder what's going on. I wonder what this means." Or, "This is interesting. Debbie is asking for a structured meal plan after our long discussion last week in which we decided that's not a good idea. I wonder what's going on."

Question the source of reluctance.
While you may think, "They don't like me," or "They think I'm stupid," clients may be reacting to you as an authority figure. They may be transferring their past difficulty with authority figures to you. For the client, cooperating may be equivalent to weakness. Resisting may be a way of making them feel strong. Clients are also reluctant in order to protect denial; they don't want to admit there's a problem. They may also be reluctant because they are having a hard day. Maybe you remind them of their mother, father or significant other. You may need to alter your approach to the situation or you may need to directly diffuse the reluctance.

Diffuse Reluctance
As mentioned earlier, it is important that reluctance is approached nonjudgmentally, and that you do not take it personally. Following are some comments that could open up reluctance to discussion:

I sense you're not wanting to try a walk this week. Am I right?

It seems like you are having a hard time talking right now. I wonder what is going on.

You're agreeing to try this new food, but I have a sense you don't want to. Am I on target?

For many people, talking about food and weight can be extremely difficult. Ask clients:

How do you feel right now, talking about your food (or eating patterns)?

How does it feel to keep food records?

Deal With Reluctance
Dealing with reluctance directly is important because it communicates to the client that their feelings are heard and understood. The clinician will not pretend their feelings do not exist. They will not be ignored. Their feelings will not be ignored. The clinician can handle the feelings that the client is experiencing. When clients experience having their feelings acknowledged and handled effectively, it models how they can then acknowledge and handle their own feelings. "If the dietitian can handle my anger, I guess I can too."

Sarah, a group member, was being confronted because of her lack of progress. Initially, she denied lack of progress. As specific instances were pointed out, she became increasingly agitated. Other group members, who had backed off with the agitation, began an attempt to placate her and make her feel better...to the point where several reached out to touch and hug her. She began to cry, and as the therapist would not let go, she became angry letting out a bloodcurdling "F___ you." (Scared the group to stone silence!) The therapist did not back off nor get angry, but encouraged her to discuss her feelings. She commented later that having the therapist sit with her in pain had impacted her to the point that this experience had been the turning point in her treatment.

Other Strategies to Deal with Reluctance

When they keep saying, "Yes, but..." Note, this is a no-win situation. Comment that, "I notice you are unable to do any of my suggestions. What shall we do?" Or, "I notice that all of my suggestions seem unworkable to you. What ideas do you have?" Then allow silence. Clarify their unwillingness to change. "We have discussed many ways to explore your eating patterns, relationship with food, etc., but you say you are unable to try any of them for a variety of reasons. I wonder what that means. What do you think?" Silence. "I am wondering if this means you are not ready to look at this or to make any changes. What do you think?" Silence.

The use of silence in session has many functions, such as:

- help redirect responsibility,
- demonstrate attentiveness,
- allow issues to remain exposed (by not moving through them quickly),
- demonstrate the clinician is confident, and
- pace the session by allowing the opportunity to slow down and reflect.

Don't take or own responsibility. When clients ask, "What do you want me to do?" There is a good chance they are asking for something they can reject. Answer by giving the question back to them in some form. "I have several ideas, but I would like to hear what you think first," or "Well, what is it you would like to accomplish at this point?," or "Well, tell me what you accomplished last week, and then from there, let's figure out what to work on this week." Giving it back to them provides the opportunity for them to answer the question. Very often clients have the answer, or can be moved towards it.

If a client is well-defended..talk in the hypothetical. "I hear you're not angry that your husband was out late last night, and it did not affect your late-night eating. However, if it were true, and you ate last night because of anger, what would it mean?" She will probably continue to defend her position. Then you may want to respond, "I hear what you're saying, but let's talk hypothetically. If your eating was because of anger, what would that mean...to your program, to your eating style, to your relationship with your husband?" Please note that you may be completely off-base in pursuing this line of discussion. What may appear to be a well-defended client, actually may not be. Always watch your own motives and feelings and avoid transferring how you feel to the client (counter transference).

If they don't believe you... again, talk in the hypothetical. "Well, if it were true that being at a level 7 on the hunger scale meant that you were not physically hungry, what would that mean to you?" "If you were to believe that eating 1,200 calories causes you to binge, how might that make your life different?"

Be curious. Explore many different ideas with clients; make it a kind of adventure to discover what is happening. For instance, your clients believe they do not have a problem accepting themselves at their current size. You have a concern about this. You might say, "How would you know if there was a problem? What would you look for?" If you believe your client is not eating enough food. They think they are. You might say, "How would you know if you were not getting enough food? What signals or situations might you look for?"

Listen to your gut! Feeling anxiety in a session, getting angry, suddenly feeling excessively sleepy or feeling like you might want to scream or cry may indicate a counter transference situation. You can choose to stay with the feeling situation and explore it, or tune it out. You only have a few moments to explore the feeling situation, because you need to be present to the client. If there is no quick answer, make a mental note to bring up the situation in supervision. If it is tuned out and not dealt with, it will come back, over and over again, and most likely, significantly impair the therapeutic relationship, making it difficult for your client to move forward.

What are they really asking for?   A client might ask, "How many calories do I need?"   Again, they may mean, "Give me something to reject."   Respond with, "How many calories do you think you need?"   Usually, the client knows the answer to this question.   What are they really asking for?   They may be testing you.

For instance, a client asked how many calories she needed. The nutrition therapist responded with, "What do you think?" The client said, "I don't know," to which the therapist responded, "Well, give me a ball park, just a rough idea of what you think it might be." She continued to state that she did not possibly know. The question was reframed several times and the same answer given. She seemed to be in a "Give me something to reject" phase. So the therapist responded, pen in hand, ready to write the meal plan, "Well, let's start at about 2,400 calories..." The client immediately responded in a raised tone of voice, "No way, 1,200 calories is the maximum needed to sustain, etc., etc., etc." They discussed what happened and moved forward with a more cooperative spirit.

DECODING THE EATING PROBLEMS
Once you are comfortable with and skilled at identifying, tolerating and discussing feelings, you are ready to use these skills to help your clients decode or solve the mysteries of their relationships with food, exercise, and their bodies.

Body Focus and Weight-Related Symptoms
Moving beyond negative body thoughts is critical in the move to size acceptance, self-acceptance, and a neutralized relationship with food and body.   When clients realize that negative body thoughts have little to do with their bodies, and everything to do with their lives, they will be better equipped to move forward in the world and with themselves. Size acceptance comes more readily when one integrates the concept that fat is not a feeling and that it is actually our thoughts which make us respond negatively to our bodies. And, happily, thoughts can be changed.

Negative Body Thoughts
But the strange notion that people should fit into clothes replaced the idea, perfectly good until then, that clothes were made to fit the person (10).

"I feel so fat," or "My thighs are disgusting," or "My stomach sticks out," or "My butt is too big," and "I feel huge," are types of comments heard so often, they are rarely challenged in our culture. They seem to almost have become accepted small talk for women.   But all of these self-deprecating thoughts and comments, and many more like them, are not facts, are not feelings, and are not truths.   Unfortunately, most do not have the self-confidence or ability to challenge and move beyond these thoughts and comments.   Actually, many who have lost weight have found that these feelings and beliefs did not change. Most still feet fat.

FAT IS NOT A FEELING
The statement, "I feel 'fat' is never really about fat, even if you are a fat person." Each time a woman looks at her thighs and says, "Yuck," she is really saying, "There's something wrong with me or with what I'm feeling." We turn our bodies into metaphors for all of our bad feelings, and we find confirmation for doing so everywhere we look (16). Ninety-nine to one hundred percent of the time, fat is not a feeling. Following are ways in which you may challenge a client who feels fat.

Define Fat

Ask your client to look up the word *fat* in the dictionary. *Fat* is typically defined as an energy rich compound, the tissue that contains a high proportion of such substances; obesity, corpulence; the most desirable part (2). Identify a true feeling with the client and again ask them to look it up in a dictionary. Compare the definition of fat to the definition of the feeling.

I Feel Concrete......

Fat is no more a feeling than *concrete* is. Ask your client if they were to say, "I feel concrete, what would you mean?" Probably that their hand or foot (or derriere) is in contact with concrete. They feel it by virtue of touching it. Concrete is not a feeling, it is not an emotion, yet one can sense that concrete is present and may say, "I feel concrete." This may be a neutral experience, or may engender feelings of happiness or disgust.

The person may *feel neutral* about the sensation of concrete:
"I am rollerblading on our concrete driveway."

The person may *feel glad* about the sensation of concrete:
"Jumping out of that plane was the scariest thing I have ever done. Boy, am I glad to be standing here on this concrete pavement, no matter how hot it is."

The person may *feel disgusted* with the sensation of concrete:
"Darn, I would have to fall on the concrete and not the grass. Now I am all bloody and bruised."

The concrete itself is a neutral object. While concrete is not a feeling, it can be loaded with feelings depending on how it is viewed.

The same is true with fat. Clients may feel the impact of having a certain amount of fat on the body; for instance, they may have difficulty bending over to tie their shoes, or zipping up their pants. They may sense that fat is present; however, fat is not a feeling. Let's take this away from the emotionally charged arena of fat and move to another part of the body...hair.

"I feel hair," may mean they feel the impact or sensation of having hair on their body or they are touching hair with their hands. Again, "I feel hair," is not expressing a feeling or emotion. However, if they believe they have too much hair or their hair is unsightly, feeling the hair may illicit a reaction of disgust. When they feel hair, their reaction could immediately be, "Yuck!" So they do not feel hair, but when they are aware of the hair they feel disgusted because of what they think about it.

It is the same with fat. They may become aware of the size of their body or the fat on their body, and as a result of what they think about its size, may have a positive or negative reaction. So they do not feel fat, but when they are aware of the fat, they feel disgusted because of what they think about it.

What If You Lived In Reuben's Era?

A person's perception of an object can engender many different feelings. If this is true, then changing one's perception of the object will change the reaction to it. In order for your clients to experience this, ask them to imagine they live in Reuben's era, when fat was in style, when fat people were used as models for paintings, admired, and held in high esteem. Thin people were deemed sickly at worse and unattractive at best. What would they think of their belly (bottom, thighs, body) if they lived during this time? Most reply, "Well, it wouldn't be so bad I guess." Would they feel as though their belly was disgusting? No, probably not. Explore their thoughts and feelings as they imagine living in this era.

Decoding Body Focus: If Fat Is Not A Feeling, Then What?

The human body serves as a reliable barometer for emotions. A client may not be aware of feelings they are experiencing, but physical and/or emotional discomfort can be a signal that these feelings are present (17).

Since fat is not a feeling, what feeling is your client experiencing? There are many techniques that can be used to help decode a fat thought. However, clients will need to have a basic understanding that fat is not a feeling before they can move through the decoding process. The health care provider *MUST* believe that fat is not a feeling. If there are any doubts, *do not do this work.* (First seek supervision. Discuss these concepts with those who believe in them. Read books from the reference list.)

Theory of Expando Thighs

The Theory of Expando Thighs, Figures 8-D and 8-E, challenges fat feelings by first exploring the manner in which a person's perception of his or her body changes from moment to moment, and day to day. It then helps the client explore what might be behind the fat feeling. It is presented here as a dialogue between the clinician, John, and client, Sara.

Sara: I feel so fat.

John: Remember our discussion about fat and how it is not a feeling? Since fat is not a feeling, I am wondering what is really going on?

Sara: I have no idea. I think you are wrong in my case. I really do feel fat.

John: I'm hearing that you really do feel fat. Let me take you through *The Theory of Expando Thighs*. Have you ever awakened one morning and felt really good? Felt thinner? And you put on your thin clothes, the ones you would avoid on a bad day?

Sara: (Cautiously.) Yeah.

John: And you're riding down the road, and look down and all of a sudden your thighs appear huge?

Sara: Yeah, that's happened! (Laughing.)

John: What had happened in the past 60 minutes? You didn't actually get larger in 60 minutes; but you actually see that your thighs are bigger. It's not the meal you ate hours ago, so what is it?

Sara: I don't know, but it happens a lot.

John: Whenever this happens, you have a choice. Imagine you are at the intersection of a fork in the road. You think "I feel fat." What would be the answer to "I feel fat?"

Sara: To lose weight, diet.

John: Right. Most people respond to "I feel fat" by thinking about altering their body shape. So, you are at the fork in the road and think "I feel fat," and then think "I need to take some weight off." Then you're off and running.... "Oh my gosh, what did I have for breakfast? I ate too much for breakfast, so now I need to go on a diet, and I have a lunch date which I think I need to cancel so that I don't have to eat lunch, and for dinner....I can change dinner. Everyone is going to be there and I planned hamburgers, but maybe I'll have broiled fish instead. And, oh my gosh! Maybe I need to go for a walk; I need to...How am I going to get this weight off? I feel so fat!"

　　You are moving further and further away from the answer to the problem. And you're on a roll. Making plans to alter the shape of your body is moving you so far from what needs to be dealt with, that you are incapable of seeing the solution. You have to slow down and back up. Let's go back to the fork in the road. At the fork in the road, when you say, "I feel fat," would the words, "I feel uncomfortable," fit?

Sara: Well, yes. Whenever I feel fat, I definitely feel uncomfortable.

Figure 8-D

Theory of Expando Thighs

Developed by Karin Kratina, MA, RD

You get up one morning feeling thin. You put on your thin clothes (the ones you would avoid on a "bad" day.) You drive down the road, look down, and suddenly your thighs are **HUGE** . . . you "feel fat". You've heard fat is not a feeling, you know you didn't really gain 10 pounds in the last few hours, so what's the deal?

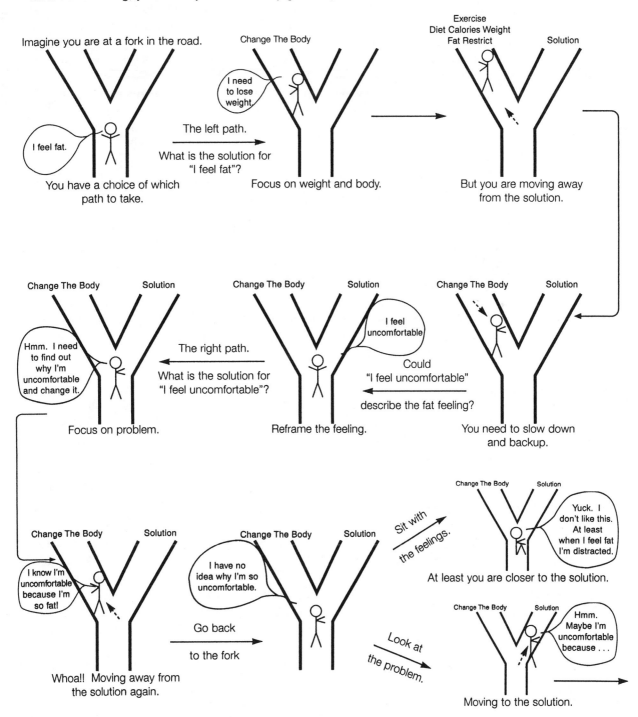

John: Okay, "I feel uncomfortable," can take the place of, "I feel fat," because whenever you feel fat, you also feel uncomfortable, right?

Sara: [Nods]

John: Okay, so we're at the fork in the road. You feel fat, which you translate as, "I feel uncomfortable." What would be the answer to, "I feel uncomfortable"?

Sara: Get comfortable?

John: I would agree with that. How would you get comfortable?

Sara: Find out what is making me uncomfortable and do something about it.

John: So, you are at the fork and trying to decide why you are so uncomfortable. I bet you say, "I'm uncomfortable because I feel so fat!" [Client laughs.] Wait a minute we're back on the path that takes us away from the solution. Let's start again at ,"I feel uncomfortable." What if you have no idea why you're uncomfortable? Sometimes you may need to choose to stay at the intersection of the fork and feel uncomfortable. However, make sure you do not begin to travel up the change-the-body path; in fact, face the other direction (to the right)!!!

You might have to feel uncomfortable for an extended period of time. Eventually, you will be able to start moving down the other road. It looks something like this... "I feel fat. No, wait a minute. Fat is not a feeling, so what am I feeling? I feel uncomfortable. Okay, good. Now, what is it that I feel uncomfortable about? Gee, I don't know, the last song on the radio reminded me of my partner. Hmm. I don't like the way he talked to me this morning. I'm really uncomfortable about that. I feel so fat and gross. Wait a minute, wrong road. Uncomfortable. Why am I so uncomfortable? Oh geez, I feel really angry at him."

A minute later: "I don't know, I feel so fat. No wait a minute, I feel uncomfortable. I'm uncomfortable because I was thinking about the fight last night. I think I need to sit down and talk with him about this."

Now you're really moving down the other path heading toward the solution from changing the body, to the solution. Moving to the solution involves identifying the feeling and deciding how to deal with it. So any time you start to say, "I feel fat," translate that into "I feel uncomfortable," and then determine the best course of action.

I'm wondering if you can relate to any part of The Theory of Expando Thighs?

What Feelings Are Stored There?

Another response to, "I feel fat," is to ask clients specifically in what part of their bodies they feel the fat. For instance, they may say they feel extremely fat in their stomach Ask them if there are feelings stored in their stomach. It is amazing how often clients can identify feelings stored in different parts of their bodies. For instance, clients might say they feel sadness in their belly. A response could be, "Then you must feel a great deal of sadness right now that's making you feel your belly is so large." If they are unable to identify the feeling stored there, ask them hypothetically. If the reason your stomach felt so big was actually because feelings were stored there, what feelings would you guess were there? For example,

Terry was a 5'4", 120 pounds, 18 year old woman who was just entering college. She frequently complained about feeling fat, and having a large bottom. Even with her weight low, she felt her bottom was out of shape and flabby. She felt she'd be happy with her body if she could tone up her bottom. She was a compulsive exerciser, and spent 6 or 7 hours a day walking and 30 to 40 minutes on buttock tucks to shape her lower torso. Her therapist explored the stored feelings concept, and she asked Terry what feelings she stored in her bottom. Terry realized that she stored anger there. She gradually came to look at the need to shape her lower torso as a code that she was angry about something. She was not always able to deal with the anger directly, and continued to do the exercises, but she became more willing and able to confront the anger.

Figure 8-E

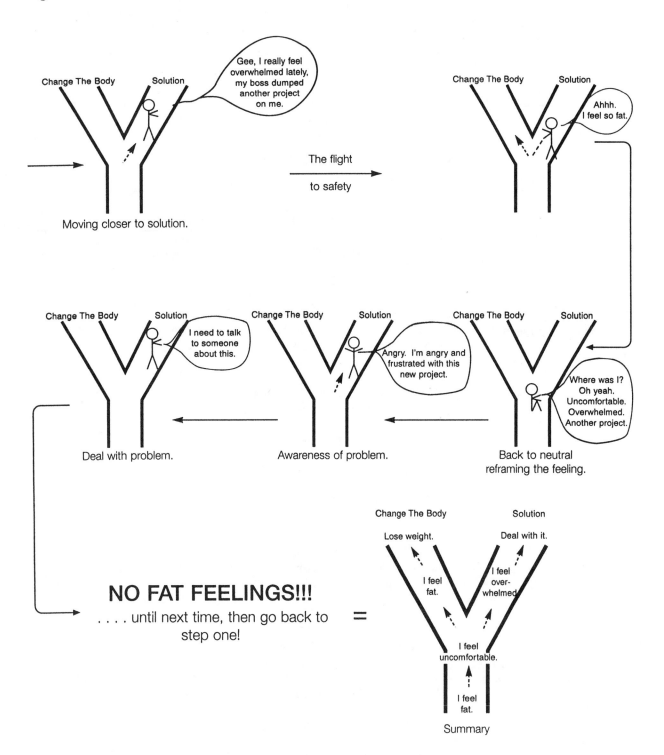

When you are on the path to the solution, you are moving further away from the need to change your body. Moving to the solution involves identifying the feeling and dealing with it. So anytime you start to say "I feel fat", translate that into "I feel uncomfortable", and determine the best course of action.

ANATOMY OF A FAT THOUGHT
The following handout, Figure 8-F, was developed by Dana Armstrong, RD, for use with her clients (18). It is based upon the work of Hirschmann and Munter (16). Walk through and explore this handout with an individual client or in a group.

Figure 8-F

ANATOMY OF A FAT THOUGHT

To begin to form a fat thought you start with

AN UNLABELED DISCOMFORT

You feel compelled to reach for food and you start

EATING

This leads to

SELF CONTEMPT
You are obsessed by a series of painful, albeit familiar thoughts about your body and your weight and how bad you are for having eaten.
Your

UNCOMFORTABLE FEELING
turns into a

FAT FEELING

You have just made the translation from

THE LANGUAGE OF FEELINGS
into

THE LANGUAGE OF FAT
The compulsive eating was a way of coping with discomfort by translating complex concerns into an obsessive preoccupation with eating and weight.
Whenever these thoughts happen, you blame your eating and your weight.

REMEMBER
You are telling the truth, but in translation.
You are referring to something else that you feel bad about.
You eat through the difficulty or yell at yourself about your size or weight, and then say the problem is fat.

WITH THIS KNOWLEDGE

You can now start to use your compulsive reach toward food as a

WAY TO BETTER UNDERSTAND YOURSELF

FOUR STEP PROCESS TO HANDLE A "BAD BODY THOUGHT"

The following outlines a four step process outlined by Hirschmann and Munter to use when a "bad body thought"(BBT) is experienced: Apologize, Challenge, Set theThought Aside, and Learn About Yourself from it (16).

Step One: Apologize

When a bad body thought occurs, slow down and use a new, internal caretaker to address it. Even before the thought is decoded, apologize to yourself for having treated yourself so badly. Bad body thoughts, after all, are abusive. (Recommend to your clients to keep track of their bad body thoughts for a specified period of time. Review these writings in session and discuss the intensity of the comments. Ask if they would ever talk to anyone else as they talk to themselves.)

Step Two: Challenge the Authority of Your Bad Body Thoughts

Use, "Who says," to challenge the beliefs behind bad body thoughts (3). Challenge the current cultural ideals that make bad body thoughts seem so normal. "...openly challenge the beliefs and assumptions behind each and every bad body thought. 'Who says that my body should look like hers?' 'Who says that my thighs are the wrong size and hers are the right size?' 'Who says my butt's too big? Who thinks so? What's wrong with large butts?' (16)."

Step Three: Set the Thought Aside

After apologizing to yourself and challenging the validity of the bad body thought, set it aside. Dismiss it.

Step Four: Learn from Your Bad Body Thoughts

Once you learn to decode them, each bad body thought can become a springboard for self-exploration. After all, each time you have a bad body thought, it means that you are ambivalent about noticing something you are thinking or feeling. Becoming adept at decoding means addressing your real thoughts and feelings with compassion and understanding, and the more compassionately you treat yourself, the less need you will have for the camouflage that bad body thoughts provide.

A WORD ABOUT THE SCALE

The weighing of clients is an increasingly controversial topic among clients and professionals alike. There are differing ideas about whether or not a client should be weighed, how often and what to do with the resulting number. Clients often allow the number on the scale to determine whether or not they will have a good day. Professionals also react to the number on the scale, occasionally with negative consequences. Professionals may:

- Weigh clients openly and comment on their weight, even when their condition has nothing to do with their weight. In this culture, this practice is, at best, extremely inappropriate, and at worse harmful. Unassuming professionals who comment about a seemingly innocuous number on the scale can unknowingly undermine ongoing treatment or cause a client to feel shame. This can make it difficult for clients to be present to, and heed the advice of the health care provider. Clients decide not to return for medical care rather than subject themselves to these embarrassments. Unfortunately, this frequently happens with the obese. We need to understand it happens regardless of a person's weight. For example,

Hannah at 5'4" and 96 pounds was a 36 year old housewife returning for a follow-up visit to a physician for a broken arm. When the nurse weighed her, she heartily congratulated Hannah on a 2 pound weight increase. Hannah was mortified and promptly set out to lose the 2 pounds, and more if she could. The therapist called the nurse to ask that she make NO comments whatsoever about Hannah's weight explaining the sensitive nature of the topic. The nurse explained she was just trying to encourage Hannah, and thought it ridiculous to not comment. It took Hannah 3 weeks to move beyond this issue.

- Comment on clients' weight after someone else has weighed them. Again, all of the above can occur.
- Weigh them with no comment. Weight is treated as just another piece of information gathered along with heart rate, blood pressure, blood lab values and urinalysis. Just as a nurse wouldn't generally comment about the appearance of urine, so do they not comment on weight.
- Weigh them blindly. The client can be weighed with their back to the scale or their eyes closed. This option is rarely offered.
- Not weigh the client. More often, professionals are finding they have no need to know a client's weight. Allen King, MD, an endocrinologist, and Dana Armstrong, RD, are among those who feel that any weighing is inappropriate. Indeed, King and Armstrong work in a very large practice treating diabetics successfully usually without knowing their client's weights (19).

To Weigh or Not To Weigh
Body weight is such a loaded issue that health care providers must take time to review the issues and determine the best course of action with each individual client. When a weight is needed, for instance when anesthesia is about to be administered, the reason for the weight should be explained and an opportunity for a blind weight provided. If weight needs to be discussed, it should done so in a candid, respectful manner.

Blind weights should always be offered to clients with weight issues. Arguably, since the majority of women in our culture have weight issues, maybe it should be standard to offer all women blind weights. Whenever a blind weight is taken, the health care provider should ensure that the weight is not discussed with the client present. Additionally, the records should not be left out where the client may inadvertently see them. Some health care providers place a sticky note over the weight. If clients suddenly decide they need to know their weight, discuss why they have changed their minds and process any issues that arise. Ask again whether they still want to know their weight before providing the client with the information.

The option of never weighing a client should be considered. Given this culture's preoccupation with the scale and weight, this is becoming a more viable option. This is especially true when:
- the goal of intervention is to decrease preoccupation with eating, exercise and body weight (20);
- there is no reason to know weight when treating a specific disease process;
- the goal of intervention is improved health;
- the client has weight issues.

NEUTRALIZE THE SCALE AND THE NUMBER
Whether or not you weigh a client, your goal should always be to neutralize the power of the scale and weight. Avoiding the scale may not necessarily do this, although avoiding it for an extended period of time can help with the process. Regardless, it is possible to bring a client to a place wherein getting weighed or not weighed is no longer a life-changing event.

Some clients may not be able to completely neutralize the scale and the number. Reassure them that this is okay. In our fat phobic, weight obsessed culture, this is very hard to do. If they do react to a number, help them learn to reframe the situation in more realistic terms. A phrase comes to mind…"Everyone deserves a first reaction, it is what they do with that reaction that counts."

Using the Scale and The Number
Of course, the number on the scale can be used in treatment to challenge cognitive distortions. There are many ways to do this. For example, prior to weighing a client, ask what they believe happened to their

weight and why they think this. Compare that to the actual weight and process with the client. This comparison can also be done in more general terms when your client has opted for a blind weight.

Weight can be used when refining hunger/satiety work. For instance, clients might be losing weight while it appears they are responding accurately to hunger/satiety signals. An analysis of the food diary shows they are consuming approximately 1,800 calories each day. You would need to look at how quickly they are losing weight, and determine if the weight is being lost naturally as their bodies move toward the set point weight or if they are actually restricting. Another option is they are not responding accurately to their hunger and satiety cues and actually restricting their intake. In these situations the weight is simply a piece of information used to help reach goals. As a rough guideline, if a client is consuming under 2,000 calories per day and losing over a 1/4 pound per week, he or she may not be eating enough food. If the scale is being used in this manner, substantial work will need to be undertaken to neutralize the impact of the numbers on the scale.

If a client is being weighed in session, allow adequate time to process the client's reaction. It is recommended clients be weighed towards the beginning of the session and they are always given the opportunity to not weigh. If they do not weigh, process this in session also. "I am wondering if there is anything going on that would cause you to choose not to weigh today." Some practitioners ask that the client wait until the beginning of the next session if they later decide to be weighed.

DECODING EATING EXPERIENCES
The following describe situations in which a client's relationship with his or her food is decoded. They are intended to demonstrate some of the techniques previously mentioned.

Decoding Nonphysical "Hunger"
Clients may indicate they feel "extremely" hungry after having eaten an amount of food that would cause them to be full. The clinician may be able to help them slow down enough to notice they are actually a 7 on the hunger/satiety scale. The health care provider could then ask, "Since 7 on the hunger scale is moderately full, and it seems you have eaten enough food to reach that fullness level, why is it that you still feel hungry?" Clients will usually express confusion. They may realize they could not be hungry, and yet they are sure they feel it. Explore how this desire for food could emanate from a feeling state. If the client cannot identify the feeling behind the hunger, ask open-ended questions about the hunger experience. Maintain a curious, attentive attitude as the underlying meaning is pursued.

One way to decode this hunger is to ask clients to touch the part of their body that is asking for food. Show them by touching your own lips, throat, heart, stomach, etc. The area from which they are feeling "hunger" can be indicative of certain feelings they are experiencing (17).

While each client is different, there are some commonalties within the experience of nonphysical hunger. If a client were to touch her or his lips saying hunger emanates from that area, the feelings to explore [may] include sadness or the desire to be nurtured. Hunger experienced in the jaw area may be indicative of feelings of frustration, stress, or anger. Hunger may be experienced in the throat area, possibly spreading into the chest. Clients may describe feeling as though they need to have food pass through this area. This hunger can often be correlated with feeling powerless and out of control in their life. This can also be indicative of attempting to suppress feelings, keeping them from coming up and/or an inability to express themselves (17).

Each client will be different. This is not a formula to present to your client, rather it is a place for you to begin exploration. Through nonjudgmental, open-ended exploration the professional can help the client decode and understand this nonphysical hunger (17). The following vignette shows this technique.

Kim
Kim was a young woman who "loved cheese." In fact, she ate it at every meal. Assuming there was something more to her relationship with cheese, it was explored further. She insisted, "I just like cheese. I've always loved cheese, my mother says I always loved cheese." Kim seemed extremely reluctant and defended herself from the questions. When she was asked how often she thought a "normal eater" eats

food they truly love. She responded, "Every day." There was little progress by the end of the session, so it was suggested she ask five of her friends how often they eat a food they truly love. (The answer tends to surprise clients because most people do not eat foods they love every day.) The client returned the next week and said the friends she questioned ate the foods they loved daily. (The friends she chose were all eating disordered. This possibly indicated her level of reluctance to exploring this issue.) The dietitian was beginning to doubt her skills, or she thought, maybe she was wrong and her client simply loved cheese. Kim was asked to touch the part of her body where she tasted the cheese. She touched her throat. It was discussed that taste occurs on the tongue and not in the throat. Kim became flustered stating, "Oh, I really taste it on my tongue." She would not let the dietitian pursue the topic.

Several weeks later, the dietitian brought it up again. She asked, "Theoretically, if you were tasting the cheese in your throat, what would that mean?" "That I'm crazy," replied Kim, who appeared both annoyed and frightened. The dietitian processed with Kim that disordered eating symptoms do not mean one is "crazy." Rather the symptoms can be seen as survival mechanisms. She suggested Kim may have developed these symptoms as a way to take care of herself because she was not taught differently. Kim, less defensive, became more willing to pursue the issue.

Kim's experience of tasting the cheese in her throat was explored further. She began to realize she was not tasting the cheese, but enjoying the sensation of swallowing and of the cheese passing through her throat. Later, she put the pieces together. Throughout her childhood, her father would prepare snacks for her which most often consisted of cheese. Her father sat at the table with her while she was eating her snack. This was one of the few times she had her father's undivided attention. She felt loved by her father during these times. Eating cheese brought similar feelings.

Kim's immediate response was to no longer eat cheese as she wanted to eliminate emotional eating. It was discussed how her relationship with this food was "decoded." The dietitian suggested rather than eliminating the cheese, she could use her desire for cheese as an opportunity to learn something about herself. When she wanted cheese, she asked herself is she really experiencing a desire for love or nurturing? If so, she would then have a choice, receive nurturing by eating the cheese, albeit ineffectively, or seek nurturing elsewhere. Attending to her desire for cheese actually helped her get in touch with such feelings as loneliness.

Since it was unlikely that nurturing was the only reason Kim selected cheese, eating cheese for taste, enjoyment, and fuel were also explored.

Decoding Food Rituals
Robert
Robert was a 53 year old real estate developer living in Texas. He weighed over 320 pounds at 6'1" tall. Robert loved to eat; he loved to cook; he wanted everyone around him to enjoy food and the eating experience. He had the reputation of being a "big eater." He could eat one or more large size pizzas for lunch along with a salad and a quart of iced tea. When he cooked pasta, Robert prepared a 2 pound package, several pounds of Italian sausage, and a pound of bacon just for his wife, thin son, and himself. When he wanted to cut down on fat and calories, he would prepare himself a salad made of a head of iceburg lettuce, 2 or 3 large tomatoes, and several large cucumbers. To this he added half a bottle of fat free salad dressing. Robert liked volume.

During group session one evening, Robert told a story about how his family attended a big family get-together back home in New Jersey the weekend before. He described how much food was served and how the meal lasted throughout the day. All of a sudden, he became pensive and said, "You know, I learned to eat a larger volume of food back home. There it meant love, close family, and prosperity. My best memories are around big Italian family meals where everyone was encouraged you to eat more. I've been eating more every day since moving to Texas ten years ago. I didn't know why volume was so important to me until now."

James

James was a 48 year old, retired marine who had never married. He lived in the Colorado mountains near a ski resort year around with two dogs as his companions and friends. At 5'10" and 245 pounds he was steadily gaining. He began seeing a nutrition therapist for his eating issues at the suggestion of his psychotherapist, who worked with him on life choices and depression. James had always wanted to live in the mountains and to be "his own boss." He now lived as he had always dreamed, but things did not feel right.

As James became heavier, he worried about having heart problems from too much exercise at such a high altitude. Although he had never been diagnosed with any heart problems or even high cholesterol, he knew neighbors with heart problems. He believed his weight could really hurt him, so he stopped walking the dogs as far each day.

James also became self-conscious about his weight around women. He rarely dated but he enjoyed attending community events occasionally with older neighboring couples and volunteering at the local library.

The nutrition therapist interviewed James and asked him about his eating habits and preferences. They explored his typical daily routines. James was open, jovial, and thoroughly entertaining at their ensuing sessions.

Up to the fourth session, nothing indicated James had an eating problem other than evening snacking. In that session however, James turned more serious and disclosed that he had been very depressed that week due to a former friend's death. As they discussed how his eating habits were affected by his sorrow and depression, it became clear that food played a major role in how he coped. To make himself feel better, he started baking his mother's and grandmothers' favorite pastry recipes and then he ate them. Food always had been used by the women in his family to soothe and reward. To James it brought back pleasant memories and warm feelings. Baking and eating the food made him feel better.

James acknowledged that his isolation and loneliness, especially in the snowy winter, contributed to his depression. Through working with both therapists, James decided to get a part time job and renew his commitment to walking after having a complete physical by his physician. James decided he needed to become more active in community events. As he met more people, he slowly learned to depend on their friendship and caring when stressful events happened in his life. James realized that the warm feelings he got from the pastries could also come from his friendships. He continued family tradition by baking pastries when friends could share them.

Rhonda

Rhonda is a 22 year old college student and aerobics instructor. She restricts her food intake during the day, typically taking in only 25% of her day's intake by 5 p.m. At that time, she has dinner, but continues to eat, bingeing throughout the evening. When she is experiencing a great deal of stress, she will binge throughout the day and evening. While Rhonda's friends purge frequently, she does so only on occasion. Each night, after she gets ready for bed and in her pajamas, she eats a bowl of cereal, which she never considers purging.

The ritualistic nature of this was intriguing, it seemed to be significant, so the therapist brought it up frequently and Rhonda recounted this evening ritual many times. Why was it always the same thing? Rhonda replied, "I'm scared to keep the binge food inside because it's the kind of food that will make me fat. But I'm also scared to go to bed empty, because then I'll wake up hungry in the morning. When I wake up hungry I eat, and then my whole day seems out of control. If I have the cereal at bed and keep it down, I'm not hungry in the morning and don't start eating until later in the day."

Rhonda began to see that when she had needs which were unmet, she felt very lonely. She identified that when she is hungry, she has a need for food; however, she was unsure how to meet this need. Cereal seemed to be involved here so it was discussed in depth. When asked of her first memory of attraction to cereal, she replied with a look of inspiration, "My mom and I used to have cereal at bedtime before she went to work the graveyard shift. This hour together seemed like the only time our schedules overlapped. After we had eaten cereal and brushed our teeth, she would tuck me into bed. It almost became a sacred ritual, so it never occurred to me to throw up the cereal. It seems as though the cereal 'tucked me in.' Whenever my mom tucked me in nice and snug, I didn't want to mess up the covers or loosen the snugness of the covers around me."

Although Rhonda now shares an apartment with one roommate, she feels alone much of the time. Her restriction and bingeing divert attention from friendships. She identified significant loneliness late at night, especially after bingeing. It seemed as though eating cereal before bed served as a powerful connection with her mother and eased her loneliness. It was decided that when Rhonda desired cereal, she would call her mother before bed and chat briefly about her day, tell her mother to sleep well, and express her love. She would then decide whether to have the cereal after she hangs up. For the first three weeks, she only felt the need to call her mother twice, and each time decided against having cereal. She reported feeling less lonely, as well as calmer and more connected with her mother and herself.

Decoding Food Selection
Ann

Ann was a 43 year old woman who had been in therapy for four years. She described her eating as "anesthetizing and numbing." To Ann food was "better than taking drugs." Ann was extremely defended when talking about her food; in fact she told her therapist that talking about food was more difficult than talking about past abuse issues. Over and over again, Ann reported her out-of-control eating episodes to the therapist. Each binge began around 9:00 in the evening when Ann would go to the kitchen and set out all the food she intended to eat on her breakfast table. She would begin eating and not move to the next food until she was finished with the first food. Methodically, she would eat all the food until she was so uncomfortable she could do nothing but lay down in bed. Ann was initially surprised at the attention the therapist paid to her eating and weight-related behaviors. Over time as the therapist maintained an open, exploring attitude without judging or pathologizing, Ann began to open up.

During this time, Ann visited a nutrition therapist who completed a nutritional assessment determining that Ann's diet was severely lacking in protein. A 24-hour recall revealed that she was taking in less than 24 grams of protein. Ann revealed she had been following this eating pattern for the past 9 or 10 years. The nutrition therapist began to explore the lack of protein in Ann's diet. Initially Ann told her that she simply did not like the taste of protein foods, e.g. meat, milk, eggs, cheese, etc. The nutrition therapist made detailed inquiry into this issue, asking Ann such questions as, when was the last time she remembers tasting specific protein foods? Did she ever like these protein foods? When was the last time she remembered enjoying them? Exactly what about them did she like or not like, was it the texture, the flavor, the smell, the sight? The nutrition therapist spent a great deal of time exploring different protein foods the same way. Ann recalled when she liked certain protein foods and what about them she had enjoyed. Eventually she revealed indirectly that she still likes some proteins, such as chicken. The nutrition therapist realized that she was not able to talk about these foods directly, and inquired about this. She asked if Ann could say the words, "I like chicken." Ann became terrified, and vehemently stated that she could not. This issue was referred to the psychotherapist.

Several weeks later, the psychotherapist asked if Ann could say those words. She became angry, but near the end of the session, agreed to say them. When she did, she began to cry and yelled, "I hate it, I hate protein, it's so...animalistic, it's so...male." Over time through work with her therapist, Ann was able to see that she had displaced many of her feelings about her childhood abuse onto food, protein in particular. She began to include more "innocuous" proteins in her daily intake, such as fat-free cheese and beans. Her health began to improve, as did her energy level. Bolstered by the positive feedback her body was giving her, Ann was able to add several other protein sources, although she still continues to avoid meat and milk products.

Decoding Relationship With Exercise
Martha
Martha, a 34 year old woman, was in therapy to deal with anxiety and relationship issues and in nutrition therapy to work on emotional eating issues. She was physically active and making progress with her food. At one point she disclosed that she had quit exercising and desired to do so. The nutrition therapist attempted to explore this, but Martha said, "I just don't want to, it's no big deal," and dismissed the subject. Whenever the topic was broached, she gave this same response. When she began to allow more exploration, the nutritionist asked, "Why don't you want to exercise?" "I don't know," she said, "I just don't want to." In response to "What comes up for you when you think about this?" she began to escalate, yelling, "F___ it, I don't care, I just don't want to!" and began to cry.

Suddenly she looked up, surprised and quit crying. She stated that a very specific memory of her bicycling after a session with her male therapist popped into her head. She felt disgusted at the memory and began putting the pieces together. Apparently, after establishing a trusting relationship with this therapist, she began to deal with sexuality issues, specifically learning to trust that she could feel sexual without having to act upon the feelings. It was after a such a session that she took a risk and allowed herself to feel sensual while exercising at his recommendation, reportedly a positive experience. Two weeks after this session, he was confronted by several of his female patients and admitted to engaging in an illicit relationship with a female patient.

Martha looked numb as she recounted this story and stated she felt that somehow the sense of betrayal and disgust she felt with the therapist had interfered with her willingness to move her body. She did not return to her active lifestyle immediately as she "couldn't make herself." She continued discussing the event and her feelings, and 4 months after this insight she began to return to her active lifestyle.

SUMMARY
Moving beyond advising to guiding is a new and challenging frontier for many health care professionals. The model of handing out advice along with food lists to change eating behaviors and create weight loss produces very limited success. The therapeutic model is not about techniques, or "fix-its," it's about relationships. Courage is needed to learn and utilize this style of counseling. Health care providers must be willing to risk mistakes to develop the necessary skills. The needed skills are difficult but the potential benefits for the client makes the effort to add these skills rewarding and worthwhile.

RESOURCES: COUNSELING SKILLS

Eating Disorders: Nutrition Therapy in the Recovery Process. Reiff D, Reiff K. Gaithersburg, MD: Aspen Publishers Inc.; 1992.
This comprehensive resource provides tools and discusses treatment techniques for eating disorders. The discussion of topics ranges from advice on establishing a multidisciplinary team to consequences of restricting food intake to laxative abuse. Includes 24 client handouts.

Nutrition Therapy: Advanced Counseling Skills. Helm K, Klawitter B. Lake Dallas, TX: Helm Seminars, Publishing; 1995. 817-497-3558.
Thirty-six highly qualified practitioners share their practical skills and years of knowledge in *Nutrition Therapy,* discussing counseling strategies and business skills. The book challenges readers to try new "helping" and counseling skills, as well as gives role models for nutrition therapy.

The Language of Feelings. Viscott D. New York, NY: PocketBooks, 1976.
Written for the general public, this book can be extremely useful for professionals. Viscott's thesis is that the language of feelings is the means by which we relate with ourselves and we need this to

ORGANIZATIONS

National Eating Disorders Organization (NEDO): 918-491-4044

The Association for the Health Enhancement of Large Persons (AHELP): 800-572-3120

The International Association of Eating Disorder Professionals (IADEP): 407-338-6494

The Nutrition Therapists subunit of the Nutrition Entrepreneurs Practice Group of The American Dietetic Association. For information call: 800-877-1600.

The Renfrew Foundation Conference: 800-RENFREW.

The Sports, Cardiovascular and Wellness Nutritionists Practice Group of The American Dietetic Association: 303-860-9418, 800-877-1600.

REFERENCES

1. Gearity A. *Attachment theory and real life: How to make ideas work.* Early Report, University of Minnesota, College of Education and Human Development, Minneapolis, MN. 1966;23:1,4-5.
2. *Webster's New Riverside Dictionary.* New York, NY: Berkley Books; 1984.
3. Reiff D, Reiff K. *Eating Disorders: Nutrition Therapy in the Recovery Process.* Gaithersburg, MD: Aspen Publishers, Inc.; 1992.
4. Kronberg S, Kratina K. The value of supervision: Part II. SCAN's *PULSE.* 1997; 16(1): in press.
5. King NL, Kratina KM. *Student Fact Sheet Series: The Disordered Eating Fact Sheet.* Chicago, IL: American Dietetic Association; Sports, Cardiovascular and Wellness Nutritionists; 1995.
6. Kratina KM, Albers MM, Myers R. Eating Disorders. In: Guyers L, ed: *Handbook of Medical Nutrition Therapy: The Florida Diet Manual.* Tallahassee, FL: Florida Dietetic Association, Inc.; 1995.
7. Helm K, Klawitter B, eds. *Nutrition Therapy: Advanced Counseling Skills.* Lake Dallas, TX: Helm Seminars; 1995.
8. Lafavi B, Kratina K. "Connection in the therapeutic relationship." SCAN's *PULSE.* 1996; 15 (2): 5-6.
9. Ornish D. *Reversing Heart Disease.* New York, NY: Ballantine Books; 1992.
10. Bloom C, Gitter A, Gutwill S, Kogel L, Zaphiropoulos L. *Eating Problems: A Feminist Psychoanalytic Treatment Model.* New York, NY: BasicBook; 1994.
11. Viscott D. *The Language of Feelings.* New York, NY: Pocket Books; 1976.
12. Kronberg S. "The value of supervision." *SCAN'S PULSE.* 1996; 15(4): in press.
13. Stuart M, Simko M. A technique for incorporating psychological principles into the nutrition counseling of clients. *Topics in Clin Nutr.* 1991; 6(4): 32-39.
14. White F, White T. Appropriate expression of feelings form. Treating Overweight and Emotional Eating Disorders. Santa Barbara, CA: Handouts from Workshop: September, 1994.
15. McTee K. Letters to the editor. *Radiance: The Magazine For Large Women.* 1995; Fall:13.
16. Hirschmann JR, Munter, CH. *When Women Stop Hating Their Bodies.* New York, NY: Ballantine Book; 1995.
17. Kratina KM, King NL. Hunger and satiety: Helping clients get in touch with body signals. *Hlthy Wt J.* 1996; 10(4): 68-71.
18. Armstrong D. Anatomy of A Fat Thought. Santa Barbara, CA: Handout from Workshop; September, 1994.
19. Armstrong D, King A. "Demand feeding" as diabetes treatment. *Obes and Hlth.* 1993; 7: 109-110, 115.
20. Carrier KM, Steinhardt MA, Bowman M. Rethinking traditional weight management programs: A 3-year follow-up evaluation of a new approach. *J Psych.* 1993; 128(5): 517-535.

9
Concepts in Action

> *Chronic dieting, paradoxically, strips [individuals] of the capacity for making self-determined, healthful choices about food and their nutrition. Dieting is not about good health. It is about ill health. Dieting is a disorder in itself (1).*

MOVING AWAY FROM DIETS

Moving Away From Diets has made it clear that while most people believe dieting is about body size, in reality, it is about a multitude of feelings. The feelings, thanks to our fat phobic and diet addicted culture, are translated into a language of fat, food, and a person's body. The diet has become the unchallenged answer. The dieter learns to eat according to rules that disregard internal signals of hunger and satiety and loses touch with these critical and trustworthy signals. They no longer trust themselves around food. "More and more, [they feel] the need for a diet and a diet surveillance group (2)."

The sense of personal failure that results is not limited to the eating environment. When there is a lack of security and safety in something as basic as the ability to feed oneself, loss of trust in oneself is inevitable. The dieter comes to see himself or herself as unreliable, untrustworthy, and insatiable in areas far beyond food and eating.

It is clear that moving beyond dieting is a complex, intensive process. *Moving Away From Diets* outlined the four primary areas that must be processed: total health orientation instead of ideal weight, eating well based on internal cues, self-acceptance, and returning to the joy of movement. The health professional has been provided tools and techniques to aid this process.

This chapter will allow the reader to see more of these concepts in action and to practice them. Remember:

- Do not assume size dictates treatment. There will be large individuals who are healthy and self-accepting who will not need to move beyond diets; there will be thin individuals who desperately need this work.
- It is imperative that the clinician be clear about their own issues in order to provide nonjudgmental assessment and treatment for clients.

REVIEW OF CLIENT FOOD JOURNALS

Following are case studies outlining a variety of eating styles. The case studies are followed by diaries and the reader is prompted to answer several questions about either a single diary or a group of diaries. These are excellent tools to take to supervision groups or explore with a colleague. There are no right or wrong answers to the questions. The authors' response to Fred's first Food Journal can be used for comparison.

The following cases are presented:
    1) Fred
    2) Connie
    3) Harriett

Fred

Fred is a 35 year old man who began dieting at the age of 12, when his mother took him to Weight Watchers because the doctor said he was, "too chubby." He has dieted on and off ever since. He is currently 5'8" and weighs 230 pounds. His lowest adult weight was 172 pounds at age 26 after a liquid weight loss diet in which he lost 68 pounds. He maintained the loss for approximately 6 months by maintaining a 1,500 calorie diet and exercising between 7 and 10 hours a week. Eventually, he was no longer able to maintain this vigilance and began to eat more, and with the same exercise regimen, began to gain weight. He became overwhelmed by a sense of failure and began to isolate. His emotional eating, typically controlled when following a strict diet or fasting during the day, was out of control. His weight reached a high of 260 pounds, at which point he began psychotherapy and was introduced to a nondiet approach. Initially, he resisted giving up dieting, believing himself to be unacceptable and unhealthy at his weight. He underwent two more diets with a combined loss of 29 pounds and gain of 36 pounds, at which point he "gave up" and committed to a nondiet approach. He was 29 years old and weighed 267 pounds. He was clinically depressed, self-rejecting, eating emotionally, and obsessed with food. He felt he could not trust himself, so he tried to follow a 1,500 calorie meal plan, which he believed was, "more than enough food." He often gorged at night.

Fred was referred to a nutrition therapist who determined his evening binges averaged 1,600 calories and were primarily deprivation-driven eating. The assessment revealed he was minimally in touch with hunger and satiety cues, and had no idea how to eat without a meal plan. His chaotic eating style made it extremely difficult to get in touch with hunger and satiety. Since he had no concept of how much he should be eating, he was given a 2,200 calorie meal plan based on the Core Minimum (see Chapter 6). Within three months, Fred was in touch with and often ate according to hunger and satiety cues although he continued to binge eat on occasion. He began work on emotional eating issues. Within 1 1/2 years, he had eliminated deprivation-driven binge eating. He emotionally ate approximately 6 times a month (although this was sporadic). The team did not monitor his weight, however, a physical examination showed he weighed 255 pounds (a loss of 12 pounds in 18 months).

Although Fred attempted exercise during this time, he reported it made him think about wanting to lose weight and caused major setbacks in treatment. He began ignoring hunger signals and restricted his food in an attempt (albeit, subconsciously) to drop weight. Since he was having such a difficult time reconnecting with exercise, he was referred to a size-friendly trainer. The trainer successfully challenge many cognitive distortions regarding exercise (work previously begun by the psychotherapist and nutrition therapist). Fred was unable to do a structured exercise program without relapse, and agreed to limit his exercise. When he realized he could do less activity and still receive benefit, he began to use the stairs at work rather than the elevator, and two months later reported "feeling better" as a result. (Just to be sure, he once carried a stopwatch to determine the amount of time he exercised. He found his total amount of time spent traversing stairs was 14 minutes. A year later, he found the same distance took 9 minutes.) Six months later, bolstered by his success, he joined an exercise class for large men and met several friends. He continued to go twice a week and "wouldn't miss it for the world." Over the next 2 years, his weight dropped 25 pounds and stabilized at 230 pounds (an overall loss of 37 pounds). He has maintained this weight for 3 years.

He is now working with a nutrition therapist once every six months. The following diaries are very similar to the diaries he brought in for a follow-up session. He no longer keeps them regularly, but uses them when he is having a difficult time or prior to seeing the nutrition therapist. These were altered to better illustrate certain issues.

NOTE: **Answer the questions on the "Review of Client Food Journal" sheet following the diary. An analysis of Fred's February 4th Food Journal is made for you on page 155. Copy and use the other review sheets for self-learning and to generate discussion with colleagues or during professional supervision sessions.**

FOOD JOURNAL

NAME: Fred F.
DATE: 2-4-96
DAY: M T W Th F Sa Su

TODAY'S GOAL AND/OR AFFIRMATION:
Make plans to go to dinner with Martha over the weekend.

TIME	FOOD AND QUANTITY	DP	MP	V	G	O	HUNGER SCALE (0 1 2 3 4 5 6 7 8 9 10)	MOOD, THOUGHTS AND/OR FEELINGS
8:00	1½ cup Raisin Bran 1 cup Skim Milk 1 banana	1			3		(graphed)	Was hungry. Looking forward to day.
11:00	1 deli bagel with cream cheese				3	1	(graphed)	Having a late lunch. Something to tide me over. Very hungry today.
2:00	Reuben sandwich Handful potato chips	1	3	1	2	1	(graphed)	Wasn't as hungry as I thought I would be. I hate late lunches, is harder to figure out my food.
3:30	Nothing! :)						(graphed)	Everyone eating cake at meeting. Wasn't hungry so saved some. There was a time when I would have eaten it anyway.
5:30	Large piece of cake					6	(graphed)	Have to work late. Ugh. Am hungry.
7:30	6 oz Baked Salmon Large baked potato with 2 tsp sour cream ½ cup broccoli 1 dinner roll Tossed salad with dressing		6	1 1	4 1	2 1	(graphed)	Dinner was good. Hit the spot.
	TOTALS	2	9	4	13	11		
	RECOMMENDED	─	─	─	─	─		

HUNGER SCALE
0 = Empty
5 = Neutral
10 = Stuffed

Graph hunger level from start to end of meal

EXERCISE: Stairs!!

DP = Dairy Protein
B/MP = Bean / Meat Protein
F/V = Fruit / Vegetable
G = Grain
O = Others

Review of Client Food Journal

Please copy this sheet for each of Fred's three Food Journals. Answer the following questions.

Client: Fred
Diary Reviewed:

1. **Comment about the quantity and quality of food eaten:**

2. **If Fred were to eat like this every day, do you believe he would:**   gain,   (Circle one.)
                                                                            maintain,
                                                                            lose weight?

   Explain your answer:

3. **What changes, if any, would you recommend (quality/quantity food intake; hunger/satiety responses, etc.):**

4. **List issues you could bring up in session based on this diary:**

Review of Client Food Journal

Fred
Diary Reviewed: February 4, 1996

1. Comment on the diary.
We know Fred is in touch with and typically eats according to hunger/satiety cues, occasionally eating emotionally. It appears his eating is physically-connected, and he appears to be eating what he wants. He eats when hungry. When time comes for a late lunch he is not as hungry as usual. It seems there are no emotional issues. He does not allow himself to get too hungry, and is not eating when not hungry and stops before full.

2. If Fred were to eat like this every day, do you believe he would gain/maintain/lose weight? (Circle one.) Explain your answer:

Although he appears to be eating a large quantity of food, over 2500 calories, he is in touch with hunger/satiety cues and has been maintaining his weight. If he continued to eat according to hunger/satiety cues, he would continue to *maintain weight,* even though it seems like a large quantity.

3. What changes, if any, would you recommend (quality/quantity food intake; hunger/satiety responses, etc.):

None, unless he had a nutrition-sensitive disease. He is ready for joyful and healthful eating work. Even then, it might be best to first explore his connection with the foods (how important each food was to him on this day) before considering any changes.

4.   List issues you could bring up in session based on this diary:

If there were several diaries, skip this one looking for more pressing issues. If all diaries were like this one, explore:
   How did it feel to not eat cake when everyone else was eating it?
   How did it feel to wait until he was hungry to eat the cake?
   How in control is he at late lunch? Explore alternatives.
   What was it like to eat lunch when not very hungry?

FOOD JOURNAL

NAME: Fred F.
DATE: 2-5-96
DAY: M T W Th F Sa Su

TODAY'S GOAL AND/OR AFFIRMATION:
Find someone to go to dinner
with over the weekend.

TIME	FOOD AND QUANTITY	DP	B/ MP	F/ V	G	O	HUNGER SCALE	MOOD, THOUGHTS AND/OR FEELINGS
7³⁰	1 deli bagel with cream cheese coffee and cream				3	1 1		Bummed Martha can't go to dinner. Will call Suzanne or Diane. Hungry.
11⁰⁰	apple			1				Work is going well. Looking forward to aqua-size!
12³⁰	Hamburger and fries		3		2 2	?		
3⁰⁰	6 Cheese crackers	1			1			Not sure what food group this is, I guessed.
5⁰⁰	apple			1				→ Am hungry but don't want to eat much before working out.
7³⁰	4 oz chicken ½ c mashed potatoes 1 cup green beans		4	2	1			Am starving. Hard to decide what I want. Ate past comfortable. Ugh.
	2 rolls				2			Don't feel so good. Can't find anyone to get together with over the weekend.
9³⁰	Cake and ice cream					10		Not hungry I know. Craving something sweet.
TOTALS		1	7	4	11	13		
RECOMMENDED		-	-	-	-	-		

HUNGER SCALE: 0 1 2 3 4 5 6 7 8 9 10

0 = Empty
5 = Neutral
10 = Stuffed

Graph hunger level from start to end of meal

EXERCISE:
1 hour aqua-size

DP = Dairy Protein
B/MP = Bean / Meat Protein
F/V = Fruit / Vegetable
G = Grain
O = Others

© Copyright 1993 Karin Kratina MA, RD / Reflective Image, Inc., Publishers 1993

FOOD JOURNAL

TODAY'S GOAL AND/OR AFFIRMATION: _____

NAME: __Fred F.__

DATE: __2-6-96__

DAY: M T W Th F Sa Su

TIME	FOOD AND QUANTITY	DP	B/MP	F/V	G	O	HUNGER SCALE (0 1 2 3 4 5 6 7 8 9 10)	MOOD, THOUGHTS AND/OR FEELINGS
8:00	1 glass skim milk 1 banana	1		1				Not very hungry. Bummed.
11:00	handful of peanuts		½			?		Hungry. Craving something sweet.
12:30	Large Hot Fudge Sundae							Stuck in meeting again, hate these things. Nothing seems to get done.
3:00	Nothing							Not hungry.
6:30	2 oz turkey ½ c broccoli 1 biscuit		2	1	1			Still don't feel good. Low energy. Don't know what's going on. Not really hungry.
8:30	2 oz Skittles					1		Just wanted something sweet.
10:00	1 glass skim milk 1 pc of cake	1				6		Really blew this day. Feel so fat. Feel disgusting. Probably gained weight
TOTALS		2	2½	2	1	7+		
RECOMMENDED								

0 = Empty
5 = Neutral
10 = Stuffed

Graph hunger level from start to end of meal

EXERCISE: ∅

DP = Dairy Protein
B/MP = Bean / Meat Protein
F/V = Fruit / Vegetable
G = Grain
O = Others

Connie

Connie is a 24 year old woman who just graduated from college with a masters in Special Education. She will start working in the fall, meanwhile, she is a sales clerk in a clothing store. She is 5'3" and weighs 165 pounds She was working out at the gym with staff for two hours each day to lose weight and tone up, which she wanted to do before she began work. As she was having much difficulty, the gym trainer referred her to a dietitian.

Connie was an extreme "all or nothing" eater. When she followed a diet, she did so expertly. Whenever she went off, she binged out of control until she could "pull herself together" and get on a diet. She complained that the older she got, the harder it was to stay on a diet. She knew she had the willpower. On her first diet at age 15, she lost 47 pounds (from 152 pounds to 105 pounds) in 4 1/2 months with the aid of Weight Watchers. At age 17, again with a commercial weight loss program, she lost 55 pounds (165 down to 110 pounds). She has dieted and lost weight several times since then. Most recently, in her senior year at college, she lost 45 pounds (from 160 to 125 pounds) in 4 months. She believed a better diet was necessary and was pleased with the idea of meeting with a dietitian.

Initially, she was appalled at the idea of eating when hungry and quitting when satisfied. "I'll be as big as a house." As this was processed, she gradually began to understand the concept that it is *the head* that wants unlimited quantities of food; however, *the body* has a limited capacity to enjoy them. She became more aware that when she becomes uncomfortably full, she still wants food. She realized that her body didn't want to continue eating and be in pain, but it was her mind that wanted the distraction and pushed forward. She recalled she would have to "check-out" or "go numb" to be able to continue eating. She was hesitant, but agreed to keep a hunger/satiety journal the first week and not follow a meal plan.

The diary dated March 10, 1997 is typical of those Connie turned in the first week. At that time, Connie was pleased both with her progress and her 3 pound weight loss. The dietitian believed she was not eating enough food to warrant becoming as full as indicated on the Hunger Scale and began to explore Connie's perception of hunger and satiety:

Dialogue Between Dietitian and Connie

Dietitian:	It looks like you didn't feel much hunger last week.
Connie:	Yea, you're right, it was a great week!
Dietitian:	It looks as though you were almost following a diet.
Connie:	Well, not really, I was eating kind of what I wanted, and quitting when I was done.
Dietitian:	It looks like you took in less than 1,400 calories. What do you think of that?
Connie:	Gee, it's a little high, I was hoping to shoot for more like 1,200, but I guess it's okay.
Dietitian:	I'm thinking that 1,400 calories for you, Connie, is actually restricting.
Connie:	What do you mean? I'm too heavy as it is, it would be good for me to lose some weight.
Dietitian:	Well, this is actually like a weight-loss program right now, and I'm concerned that even though you're restricting, you're not experiencing hunger. I wonder why that is?
Connie:	Oh, I don't know, some days I'm ravenously hungry the whole day, and other days, I'm not hungry at all. It seems like charting my hunger this past week, I wasn't hungry at all.
Dietitian:	I wonder if it's when you're following a rigid diet that you don't feel much hunger?
Connie:	Well, yeah, I guess that's true. I really like it that way. It seems like what happens is that I'm not hungry at all, and then when I see the food, suddenly I feel hungry.
Dietitian:	What do you think that's about?
Connie:	I don't know, it's really scary, I don't like it. I tried to avoid food, because it seems like when I see it, I suddenly get hungry.
Dietitian:	I wonder if you have actually been hungry all along, but have not been aware of it.
Connie:	What do you mean?

Dietitian:	Well, hunger can be very subtle. If you ignore it, it will go away for a little while, and it will come back. You can use the analogy that it comes back to tap you on the shoulder, it waits, then taps again, this time a little louder. If you continue to ignore it, it quits tapping, and goes underground. Your body figures that since you're not listening to it's hunger signals, it's got to find another way to get you to eat. So it goes underground and causes you to think about food more often. You find yourself thinking about food, your weight, your diet, etc. much more often. You might find yourself heading to the cookbook section of the bookstore, picking up a *Southern Living*, reading recipes, being interested in what other people are eating, watching what other people eat at the restaurant. In general you find yourself more food-focused.
Connie:	Well, that happens to me. It seems like I think of food all the time, even when I'm not hungry. But I also this kind of general emptiness in me before meals, this emotional emptiness, and I don't know what that's about. I think I just want to eat emotionally.
Dietitian:	Can you describe that feeling for me?
Connie:	Well it's kind of a gnawing emptiness. It makes me feel kind of tired. It won't go away, it's very bothersome, I hate it.
Dietitian:	Do you ever use coffee or diet sodas to get rid of it?
Connie:	How did you know!? It works, it works almost every time, I can drink coffee or diet soda and that feeling will go away, that's how I know it's emotional.
Dietitian:	Connie, I'm beginning to wonder if that gnawing feeling that you're interpreting as emotional hunger, is not actually your physical hunger.
Connie:	How could that be? I'm not hungry. I'm only hungry when if feel out of control and then I end up bingeing. Then I'm hungry and I hate it. But I'm not hungry now, I wasn't hungry this past week.
Dietitian:	I'm wondering if you pushed your hunger underground, and as long as you could hold it underground, you're able to diet, and suddenly when you're no longer able to hold it underground, you go on a rampage, and you start bingeing?
Connie:	Well, yeah, if I could just quit bingeing, I think everything would be okay.
Dietitian:	Actually, Connie, it's the other way around. You need to pay attention to your hunger and quit restricting in order to be able to quit bingeing.
Connie:	I don't think I can do that.
Dietitian:	Well this week, I'd like to try something a little bit different with your food diary, if that's okay. I'd like you to chart what you're calling your physical hunger in one color ink, and then right below that, I'd like you to chart your emotional hunger. Does your emotional hunger change when you're eating.
Connie:	Yeah, it does, it goes away when I'm eating, but I don't think that has anything to do with the food.
Dietitian:	That's okay, what I'd like you to do is chart your physical hunger from the beginning of the meal to the end of the meal, and at the same time chart your emotional hunger from the beginning of the meal to the end of the meal.
Connie:	It sounds pretty silly, but I'll do it.

The next week Connie returned and presented her diary. Answer the questions regarding the diary dated March 17, 1995.

FOOD JOURNAL

TODAY'S GOAL AND/OR AFFIRMATION:
_____
_____

NAME: _Connie_
DATE: _3-17-96_
DAY: M T W Th F Sa (Su)

TIME	FOOD AND QUANTITY	DP	B/ MP	F/ V	G	O	HUNGER SCALE 0 1 2 3 4 5 6 7 8 9 10	MOOD, THOUGHTS AND/OR FEELINGS
8⁰⁰	1½ cup cereal 1 cup milk 1 muffin	1			3 1			Am not hungry at all. I don't like charting the "wanting" place, it's scary. It wants everything. I don't want to think about it. I can't believe I agreed to do this.
12⁰⁰	2 oz turkey on large roll lettuce & tomato 1 apple		2	1 1	2			This is stupid
6⁰⁰	2 oz fat free cheese on 1 cup pasta with sauce 1 cup broccolli	2		2	2			I feel so full and fat.

DP = Dairy Protein
B/MP = Bean / Meat Protein
F/V = Fruit / Vegetable
G = Grain
O = Others

TOTALS: 3 | 2 | 4 | 8
RECOMMENDED:

0 = Empty
5 = Neutral
10 = Stuffed

Graph hunger level from start to end of meal

EXERCISE: _1 hour weight lifting_

© Copyright 1993 Karin Kratina MA, RD / Reflective Image, Inc., Publishers 1993

FOOD JOURNAL

TODAY'S GOAL AND/OR AFFIRMATION:
_____
_____

NAME: _Connie_
DATE: _3-10-96_
DAY: M T W Th F Sa (Su)

TIME	FOOD AND QUANTITY	DP	B/ MP	F/ V	G	O	HUNGER SCALE 0 1 2 3 4 5 6 7 8 9 10	MOOD, THOUGHTS AND/OR FEELINGS
8⁰⁰	Coffee							Not hungry
9³⁰	1½c cereal 1c skim milk	1			3			Guess I should have breakfast
12³⁰	2 oz tuna with yogurt 2 slices whole wheat bread 1 apple		2	2 1				Feeling really good, not really even hungry, which is really nice. Eating because I know I should
3³⁰	1 apple			1				
6²⁰	3 oz broiled fish small baked potato ½ cup carrots		3	2 1				Good day! Feel proud of myself. Except that I probably didn't need to eat as much as I did. The dietician was right, it helps to chart my hunger! I like not being very hungry! Makes me feel good

DP = Dairy Protein
B/MP = Bean / Meat Protein
F/V = Fruit / Vegetable
G = Grain
O = Others

TOTALS: 1 | 5 | 3 | 7 | –
RECOMMENDED:

0 = Empty
5 = Neutral
10 = Stuffed

Graph hunger level from start to end of meal

EXERCISE: _1 hour treadmill_

© Copyright 1993 Karin Kratina MA, RD / Reflective Image, Inc., Publishers 1993

Review of Client Food Journal

Please copy this sheet for two of Connie's Food Journals. Answer the following questions.

Client: Connie
Diary Reviewed: March 17, 1996
              April 19, 1996

1. Comment on this dairy:

2. It appears that what Connie calls her emotional hunger is actually her physical hunger, and she negates her physical hunger by calling it a "wanting" that she sees is not okay. How would you help Connie realize her signals are confused?

3. How would you use the hunger/satiety responses to increase Connie's awareness of the gradual changes in her hunger? Or, the fact she usually tries to ignore it?

4. What changes, if any, would you recommend (quality/quantity food intake; hunger/satiety responses, etc.):

5. List issues you could bring up in session based on this diary:

Several weeks later, Connie was able to see that what she interpreted as emotional hunger was actually physical hunger. Soon after, she reported that she was not hungry again. Exploration revealed that Connie did not feel hungry until right before she was to eat, and then she felt ravenous. This made her feel out of control and she was "terrified" of her hunger.

The manner in which hunger develops was discussed. Connie realized that she interpreted hunger levels 3 and 4 as "not hungry," they didn't count. When she suddenly became aware of her hunger at a level 2, she became overwhelmed. Connie agreed to chart her hunger hourly to become aware of the progression of her hunger. It was again discussed that Connie was not eating enough food. Review the diary dated April 19, 1995.

FOOD JOURNAL

NAME: _Connie_
DATE: _April 19, 96_
DAY: M T W Th (F) Sa Su

TODAY'S GOAL AND/OR AFFIRMATION:

TIME	FOOD AND QUANTITY	DP	B/MP	F/V	G	O	HUNGER SCALE 0 1 2 3 4 5 6 7 8 9 10	MOOD, THOUGHTS AND/OR FEELINGS
7⁰⁰								
8⁰⁰	1½ cup cereal 1 cup milk 1 muffin	1			3 1			
9⁰⁰								
10⁰⁰ 11⁰⁰ 12⁰⁰ 1⁰⁰	2 oz turkey on 2 slices bread lettuce & tomato 1 apple		2	2 1				I'm feeling hungry and it is not lunch time yet, feeling out of control. Was very hungry at 1⁰⁰
2⁰⁰								
3⁰⁰ 4⁰⁰ 5⁰⁰ 5³⁰	8 oz yogurt, raisins & a banana	1		2				Hungry again. What is the matter with me? Really hungry now. I'll eat something now even though dinner is
6⁰⁰ 7⁰⁰ 7³⁰	1 large pita with 2 oz turkey, broccoli		2	2	1			at 7pm. Don't want to, but am so hungry. → Great, ate too much. Won't be hungry at dinner.
8⁰⁰ 9⁰⁰	handful pretzels				1			Overate today.

DP = Dairy Protein
B/MP = Bean / Meat Protein
F/V = Fruit / Vegetable
G = Grain
O = Others

	TOTALS	2	3	5	9	
	RECOMMENDED					

0 = Empty
5 = Neutral
10 = Stuffed

Graph hunger level from start to end of meal

EXERCISE:
Stairmaster ½ hour

Harriet

Harriet is a 43-year-old professional business woman who owns her own company. She presented with complaints of not being able to follow a diet and believed she was "too fat." She is 5'6" and weighed 145 pounds.

Her initial assessment revealed she has been on and off diets since the age of 17. She tried almost every commercial weight loss program excluding fasting programs. Her adult weight fluctuated from a high of 148 pounds to a low of 128 pounds. Her goal weight was 120 pounds and she believed she would not be satisfied until she reached it. Apparently, several weight loss programs told her she should weigh this since "I am small-boned."

Her assessment also revealed she was in touch with hunger and satiety cues. Her last diet had been 6 months prior in which she reduced her weight to 132 pounds (a 16 pound loss). Much of the assessment was focused on her history of dieting. Although she was seeking another diet, the dietitian suggested trying a nondiet approach for a while. Harriet, who was extremely frustrated, reluctantly agreed. She agreed to keep food journals focusing on her hunger and satiety.

During the initial two weeks, she frequently forgot to chart hunger and satiety, and when she did, reported she was guessing. Harriet said she "got too busy" and forgot. The dietitian processed this reluctance and revealed Harriet was fearful of slowing down long enough to pay attention to hunger and satiety. This type of work continued for the next month. Each session began with Harriet asking for a diet, ending with a discussion of her fears and renewed commitment to pay attention to her cues. Harriet realized a diet was not the answer, but she saw the alternative as completely overwhelming. Since they were not able to make progress, the dietitian referred her to a psychotherapist. At this time, it was decided Harriet would not work with the dietitian.

In therapy, significant issues regarding her ability to take care of her own needs arose. Food was a way she calmed herself. In fact, it was the only way she knew to take care of herself and soothe her anxiety. Keeping track of hunger and satiety was terrifying to her because it meant facing these issues. She frequently requested the therapist help her lose weight so she could feel better, and it took significant effort and patience for the therapist to refocus these issues. Harriet eventually began to appreciate her own unconscious efforts at taking care of herself. The therapist pursued this use of food to comfort and soothe and began to deal with underlying issues of dependency and neediness. The therapist validated the vulnerability Harriett felt when she expressed her needs and affirmed her need for self-care.

Six months later, Harriet was referred back to the dietitian. While Harriet still had fears about slowing down and taking care of herself, she felt she had the support to move forward. Although she still wanted to lose weight, she agreed to put that "on the back burner" for awhile. Within a month, she was able to consistently keep food diaries. Three days follow. Fill out only one "Review" for the three days.

FOOD JOURNAL

NAME: Harriett
DATE: 1/4/96
DAY: M T W (Th) F Sa Su

TODAY'S GOAL AND/OR AFFIRMATION:

TIME	FOOD AND QUANTITY	DP	B/MP	F/V	G	O	HUNGER SCALE (0 1 2 3 4 5 6 7 8 9 10)	MOOD, THOUGHTS AND/OR FEELINGS
8:00	2 Toaster waffles with 2T syrup / 2 pieces sausage / 1 glass skim milk / Coffee	1			2	2 / 2		Really hungry. It's distracting.
11:30	Turkey sandwich/mustard / 1 Orange / 1 pc apple pie		4	1	2	1		Pretty hungry. I like this restaurant! Concerned about project with Tom
2:00	1 bag chips + diet coke					1		Kind of hungry. This did not hit the spot. Gotta go get the kids, drop them off and finish project with Tom.
3:30	1 large cheese danish / 1 glass whole milk	1				1		Am starving. This should tide me over. Need to cook dinner, feel rushed.
6:00	Broiled chicken leg + breast / 1cup rice and butter / ½ c broccoli		8	1	2	1		Dinner was good.
10:00	Bowl ice cream and banana			1		1		Watching TV
TOTALS		2	12	3	6			
RECOMMENDED								

DP = Dairy Protein
B/MP = Bean / Meat Protein
F/V = Fruit / Vegetable
G = Grain
O = Others

0 = Empty
5 = Neutral
10 = Stuffed

Graph hunger level from start to end of meal

EXERCISE: NO TIME !!

FOOD JOURNAL

NAME: Harriett
DATE: 1/5/95
DAY: M T W Th (F) Sa Su

TODAY'S GOAL AND/OR AFFIRMATION:

TIME	FOOD AND QUANTITY	DP	B/MP	F/V	G	O	HUNGER SCALE (0 1 2 3 4 5 6 7 8 9 10)	MOOD, THOUGHTS AND/OR FEELINGS
8:00	3 egg whites scrambled with cheese / 1 deli bagel with butter and jelly / ½ cup grits / coffee	1	1½		3 / 1	1		No feelings.
12:00	2c eggplant rotitini / 2 rolls/butter / 1 salad with dressing / 1 cup frozen yogurt	2		2 / 1	2	2 / 2 / 1		Business meeting. I ate too much, I'll never lose weight. I think I need a meal plan.
3:30	bag pretzels + apple			1	1			
5:00	handful of nuts / cocktail		1			1		Going out to dinner with Keith. Am excited.
6:30	6oz flounder / 1 lg baked potato with lemon / ½ cup carrots / 1 ceasar salad		6	1 / 1	3			Ate way too much.
TOTALS		3	8½	6	12	8		
RECOMMENDED								

DP = Dairy Protein
B/MP = Bean / Meat Protein
F/V = Fruit / Vegetable
G = Grain
O = Others

0 = Empty
5 = Neutral
10 = Stuffed

Graph hunger level from start to end of meal

EXERCISE:

Review of Client Food Journal

Please evaluate all Harriett's Food Journals on one sheet. Answer the following questions.

Client: Harriet
Diaries Reviewed: January 4,6,7, 1996

1. **Comment on this dairy:**

2. **Does it appear Harriet is in touch and eating according to hunger/satiety cues? Explain:**

3. **If Harriet were to eat like this every day, do you believe she would:**
gain, maintain, or lose weight? (Circle one)

Explain your answer:

4. **Comment on her relationship with hunger. How would you address these issues in session (quality/quantity food intake; hunger/satiety responses, etc.):**

5. **List issues you could bring up in session based on this diary:**

6. **Harriett still has some focus on weight loss and looking for a meal plan. How would you redirect her based upon the information on these diaries?**

FOOD JOURNAL

NAME: Harriett
DATE: 1/6/96
DAY: M T W Th F Sa Su

TODAY'S GOAL AND/OR AFFIRMATION:

TIME	FOOD AND QUANTITY	DP	B/ MP	F/ V	G	O	HUNGER SCALE 0 1 2 3 4 5 6 7 8 9 10	MOOD, THOUGHTS AND/OR FEELINGS
8:00	2 cup cereal 1 cup skim milk 2 sl toast with low fat butter	1			4 2	 2		Really hungry. In a good mood. Had fun last night.
11:00	1 bagel with nonfat cream cheese				3	1		Lunch is late today
12:45	Ham and Cheese Sandwich / mustard Chips, low fat	1	3	1	2	 1		Eating at desk. Rushed.
2:00	Bag pretzels				1			Doing good, all low fat so far.
4:30	Apple with low fat peanut butter		1	1				Feeling good about my food today.
6:00	2 cup pasta with 3/4 cup meat sauce 2 dinner rolls (no butter!) Salad and a little dressing		2	 1	4 2	 1		Eating with family. Eating good foods.
9:00	cup icecream (non-fat) 4 cookies				1	1 4		I'm trying to do low fat, but I need more structure. This is not working.
	TOTALS	2	6	3	18	10		
	RECOMMENDED							

DP = Dairy Protein
B/MP = Bean / Meat Protein
F/V = Fruit / Vegetable
G = Grain
O = Others

0 = Empty
5 = Neutral
10 = Stuffed

Graph hunger level from start to end of meal

EXERCISE:

REFERENCES

1. Bloom C, Gitter A, Gutwill S, Kogel L, Zaphiropoulos L. *Eating Problems: A Feminist Psychoanalytic Treatment Model.* New York, NY: BasicBooks; 1994.

2. *Size Acceptance & Self-Acceptance. The NAAFA Workbook: A Complete Study Guide.* 2nd Edition. Sacramento, CA: NAAFA; 1995.

10
Marketing the Nondiet Approach

MARKETING IDEAS

Getting publicity for a program or service is a snap if you have a large advertising budget. Few of us have that luxury today. Fortunately there are lots of ways to get (almost) free publicity for your nondiet program. Many options entail spending more time than spending dollars, but they usually pay-off with big dividends after you begin investing regularly.

Here are ten easy ways that you can invest wisely, not expensively, in marketing:

1. *Research your market.* Learn what nondiet programs or services already exist in your community. Talk to other professionals who work with weight, food, and self-esteem issues. Organize a focus group from the public of diet "causalities" and discuss their needs in order to gain information and support.

2. *Seek out referrals.* Use your existing connections to invite referrals for the nondiet approach. Satisfied clients are always your best referral sources. Other professionals can also provide referrals, so keep them up-to-date on your services with letters, newsletters, and copies of nondiet articles.

3. *Network, network, network.* Develop new connections by joining professional and community organizations where you may meet new clients or like-minded professionals. Get out of your usual "sphere of influence" and consider completely different group settings.

4. *Create an image.* Let your business cards and stationary accurately reflect you and the nondiet image that you want to portray. Use color and artwork to add nonverbal cues about your message. Give out your business cards in doubles--one for the recipient and one for a friend.

5. *Let your voice mail do the talking.* Make the most of your voice mail system and let it function as a marketing tool when you are not personally available. Be brief, provide a concise description of your services, and personalize your message with positive nondiet tips for your callers.

6. *Get involved in your community.* Participation in community events is a satisfying way to increase your visibility and raise the profile of your services. Plan or cosponsor activities which promote positive nondiet messages like a celebration of International No-Diet Diet Day or Eating Disorder Awareness Week.

7. *Write, write, write.* Share nondiet messages via the written word in: press releases about your services to the media; letters to the editor about current community issues related to nutrition, health and fitness; and, motivational articles for local newspapers, newsletters or magazines.

8. *Speak or teach.* Public speaking enhances your credibility, increases your exposure, and polishes your image--and you can make contact with lots of potential clients and customers at the same time. Offer a taste of the nondiet approach in presentations to professional groups or teach a community class.

9. *Surf the net.* Electronic communication can help you connect with clients and colleagues in town, across the country, and around the globe. Check online forums to track the latest trends, observe your competitors, preview hot products, and investigate the latest scientific research.

10. *Always exceed expectations.* Look for quick and easy ways to add value to your services. Give clients a little more than they expect in terms of quality, quantity, and response time. Always give a little extra without giving it all away!

MEDIA RELATIONS: How can you spread the nondiet message in the media?
Programs, like your nondiet programs, are always looking for exposure. Newspapers, television channels and radio stations are always looking for news. They want the local angles on national stories as well as good news about community activities. Nondiet programs offer ideal opportunities for win-win media relations. Your program gets the positive publicity it needs and the media gets a good story for its local audience.

Food and health issues have been, and will continue to be, hot topics in the media. A local nondiet or fitness event can help the media provide a local angle on national food and nutrition stories like:
- the dangers of chronic dieting;
- the epidemic of eating disorders in the United States;
- the pleasure principle in health promotion programs; or,
- encouraging activity for children and teens.

You're also likely to get great publicity if you can tie a local event into a bigger celebration like: National Nutrition Month in March, International No-Diet Day (May 6th), and National 5 a Day Week in September, to name a few options.

Developing a positive, long-term relationship with the media is a lot easier than you might think. Here are five pointers for successful media relations--quick tips for getting the publicity that the nondiet message deserves.

1. Find the right person. Make sure that you have the correct spelling of a reporter's name, as well as appropriate address, telephone, and fax number.
2. Think like a reporter. Give reporters what they need, when they need it. Make their jobs easy and you'll get plenty of coverage for your activities.
3. Make it simple, make it positive, make it fun. Consumers are confused and tired of hearing what they shouldn't eat. They want to hear what they can eat.
4. Be available. Put your name, telephone and fax number on everything you send to the media so that it is always easy for them to contact you.
5. Be persistent. Remember that it takes time to develop a relationship with the media. If your first story isn't covered, try, try again.

GROUPS IDEAS: How can you present the nondiet approach to a group?
Nondiet messages can be easily incorporated into any nutrition or fitness groups or community programs. More intensive workshops and small group sessions are also popular (see outlines for one day, four week and eight week formats). Groups offer additional benefits compared to individual sessions. For example, in groups, participants receive:

- more information and interaction at a lower cost for participants,
- increased support from other people in a similar situation,
- repeated reinforcement of nondiet concepts and messages,
- more opportunities to hear about varied obstacles and how to deal with resistance to change,
- more revenue potential per hour.

Groups are probably most powerful when they utilize a team training model, that is several professional and peer presenters with a consistent message and different teaching styles. Effective teams involve some combination of:

- Nutrition experts (registered dietitian/nutrition therapist)
- Mental health professionals (psychologist, counselor, social worker, or art therapist)
- Movement specialists (fitness instructor, exercise physiologist, dancer, yoga teacher, physical therapist, or movement therapist)
- Health care provider (physician, physician assistant, nurse, or nurse practitioner)
- Fashion consultant (model, clothing designer or image consultant)

As a facilitator, you can add excitement, interest, and value to group interactions by doing more than just talking. Adult learners are more committed, successful, and satisfied when they have fun and get information in several different ways. Lecture, discussion and question-answer sessions are only a few of the teaching techniques that can be used to share nondiet messages. Consider adding pizzazz to a nondiet group with one or more of the following:

- Music (as background, for setting mood, and to inspire movement)
- Food (for meals, snacks, and experiential learning)
- Art (to look at, to make, and to share)
- Fashion (clothes, shoes, accessories, jewelry, make-up, and hair)

The location of group meetings deserves careful consideration. The setting must be easily accessible, as well as safe and comfortable. Some possibilities include:

- women's center, YWCA, or community center,
- hospital, medical center, clinic, or other health care facility,
- fitness facility, health club, or yoga center.

SUMMARY

The timing is right for the nondiet approach. The public is burned out on diets, weary of drugs and expensive alternatives that demand a person's dependence to be successful. Look around your community and assess the competition, identify their weak points, develop messages that play to your strong points, and create a strong presence for your program in the marketplace.

Following are sample promotional items that will illustrate successful programming concepts and ideas.

Sample Program: One-Day Workshop

Body Trust:
Undieting Your Way to Health & Happiness

8:30 am   Registration and Coffee

9:30 am   You are not the problem -- Dayle Hayes, MS, RD
Most women blame themselves for their dieting "failures," but, in reality, it is diets that are the problem. We'll talk about the diet/binge/gain cycle and explore successful ways to "undiet."

10:00 am Loving your body -- Gayle Williams, MS, LPC
Women grow up believing society's myths about weight and body shape. By freeing yourself from the myths and negative attitudes (fatism), you can learn to trust your body again.

11:00am Mirror Image-- Sandra Ottman
Feeling bad about their bodies make women both unhappy and unhealthy. We will share easy ways to begin to love the body you have, to give up the beauty myth, and to reclaim your own inner strength.

12:00 noon   Buffet Lunch

1:00 pm   Feeding Your Body -- Dayle Hayes, MS, RD
Undieting means learning to tell the difference between physical hunger and other needs (both emotional and physical), and having permission to enjoy all foods. By undieting, you can learn to eat what, when, and only as much as your body needs.

2:00 pm   Moving Your Body -- Dayle, Gayle and Sandra
The rules and shoulds about exercise keep many women from enjoying the benefits of physical activity. You will learn the secrets of gentle, safe and pleasurable activity.

2:30 pm   Nurturing the Trust -- Dayle, Gayle and Sandra
Trusting and loving your body in a fat phobic world isn't easy. The workshop leaders will share practical strategies for integrating this new approach into all aspects of your daily life.

3:30 pm   Workshop Ends

Body Trust:
Undieting Your Way to Health & Happiness

Sample Program: Four-Week Follow-up Group

Session I   **Self-Acceptance**
- freeing yourself from prejudices against fat
- grieving the loss of the "thin" fantasy
- transforming body image

Session 2   **Stomach Hunger**
- legalizing food
- ending deprivation
- learning to feed yourself on demand

Session 3   **Mouth Hunger**
- sorting out food cravings and emotions
- legalizing and accepting feelings
- assuming responsibility for your emotional self

Session 4   **The Diet/Binge Cycle**
- understanding fat thoughts
- learning not to yell at yourself
- breaking the links

Sample Program: Eight-Week Follow-up Group

Session 1   **Back-to-basics**

Session 2   **Getting in touch I: Stomach hunger**

Session 3   **Getting in touch II: Mouth hunger**

Session 4   **Self-talk & self-esteem**

Session 5   **Trust your body & nutrition**

Session 6   **Loving yourself & self-care**

Session 7   **Body image & the beauty myth**

Session 8   **Putting it all together**

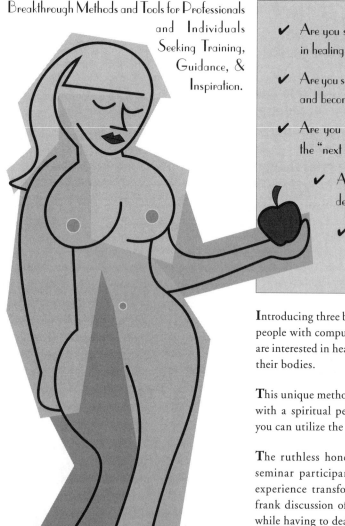